Introduction to

EXERCISE SCIENCE

Pauline Entin

Department of Biological Sciences, Northern Arizona University

J. Richard Coast

Department of Biological Sciences, Northern Arizona University

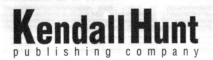

Kendall Hunt
publishing company

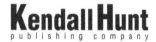

www.kendallhunt.com
Send all inquiries to:
4050 Westmark Drive
Dubuque, IA   52004-1840

TABLE OF CONTENTS

Chapter 1

INTRODUCTION

What Is Exercise Science?

Exercise science is the study of how the body performs exercise and responds to exercise. This sounds like a very broad description, but exercise science is a broad field. It encompasses anatomy, physiology, mechanics, psychology, and neurobiology as those areas relate to the evaluation of exercise, human performance, and ways to improve our health through exercise. With the world-wide increase in the number of people who are overweight or obese and the number of people with diabetes, exercise is in the forefront of preventive health care.

Exercise science has a number of subdivisions in it (Figure 1–1). These address the areas mentioned above. Specifically, exercise science includes the fields of Exercise Physiology, Kinesiology and Biomechanics, Motor Behavior, Clinical Exercise Physiology, Sports Psychology and Sociology, and more recently, Health and Wellness. The terms used to describe these fields may differ slightly between texts and institutions, but all of these areas are included under the broad umbrella of exercise science.

Exercise Physiology is the study of how the body systems respond to both acute (one bout) and chronic (over time, also referred to as training) exercise. In this field we examine the metabolic, musculoskeletal, cardiovascular, respiratory, and endocrine systems in depth, and to a lesser extent, the neural, gastrointestinal, and renal systems and how they respond to exercise.

Kinesiology, or Functional Anatomy, and Biomechanics are the study of the anatomy and mechanics of movement. This can involve the muscles and forces seen in throwing and running, or the actions of external forces on the body in such activities as a football tackle, or even an automobile accident.

Motor Behavior is a combination of the disciplines of motor control, motor learning, and motor development. Motor control is how the brain, nerves, and muscles combine to initiate and detect movement. Motor learning is the study of how we learn tasks that involve movement. Motor development researchers study how we acquire movement skills as we mature and as we age.

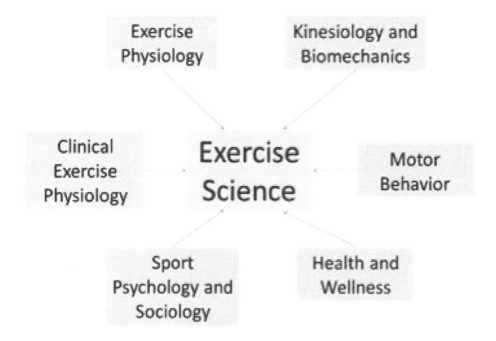

FIGURE 1–1. Exercise science and its subdisciplines.

Clinical Exercise Physiology is a branch of exercise physiology that deals specifically with exercise and training in people with diseases or disabilities. Predominantly, it emphasizes exercise in people with heart disease, the number one killer of adults in developed countries. Increasingly, there is also a focus on the overweight and obese population.

Sport or Exercise Psychology is the study of the effects of exercise on our mental processes, as well as the ways our mental processes affect our sport or exercise performance. Sport Sociologists study the role of sport and exercise in society, such as how sports reflect our cultural beliefs and values. Examples of this include the role of women in sports, or the effect of exercise on the population.

Finally, Health and Wellness, or Fitness and Wellness, examines how exercise improves physical, mental, social, and intellectual well-being. For example, exercise has a role in reducing obesity and type 2 diabetes. This field is not as well defined as some of the others, but, in many ways, may be one of the most important in exercise science as it addresses issues such as health care and the role of exercise within the health care arena.

As you should be able to see from the previous paragraphs, in order to truly understand the field of exercise science, background study in other areas is critical. Therefore, most exercise science programs have prerequisites including anatomy and physiology, physics, chemistry, and psychology. The understanding gained in these courses is the critical foundation for the courses in an exercise science program.

Where Did Exercise Science Come From?

The field of exercise science is constantly changing and evolving. Most people see the recent history of exercise science and view the field as having diverged from physical education, and indeed, to some extent, this is true. Within the last 20 years, many exercise science programs have emerged from physical education or kinesiology and have become independent, or have merged with other programs such as biology or nutrition. However, exercise science has a much longer and varied history than simply coming from physical education programs. At the turn of the previous century, the bases of exercise science were in medical and ergonomic programs. Ergonomists study ways, among other things, to improve work performance or efficiency in the workplace. In order to do this, an ergonomist must understand how the body functions and under what conditions it functions best—just like we do in exercise science. Now, ergonomics is taught mainly out of colleges of Engineering in programs such as Human Factors. Many physicians were also interested in exercise as a way of decreasing the incidence of disease. Traditionally, exercise was not a large part of a physician's training, but it has increased with the increase in the incidence of obesity and diseases that accompany a sedentary lifestyle. In fact, the American Medical Association (AMA) and the American College of Sports Medicine (ACSM) have jointly fostered a program termed Exercise Is Medicine™, which, in one of its roles, advocates for training of physicians and other health care professionals in exercise.

Research Basics for the Sciences

In any scientific field, being able to perform, analyze, and read about studies is critical. Scientific studies are the basis for our knowledge and practice in exercise science. Reliance on evidence garnered from properly interpreted scientific studies is what separates simply having an opinion on a topic from having an informed idea of the background and what is true and what is not true about a question. Examples of the importance of using scientific studies are the many diets that are available to people. Questions that are debated, not only in the scientific literature, but in the news outlets and in the blogosphere include those around the high vs. low carbohydrate diet, various drugs, both prescription and over-the-counter, that may/may not cause us to lose weight, the idea that one can safely lose twenty pounds in a month, miracle weight loss foods, and many others. While a person can get initial information on a question from websites and general interest magazines, in order to truly be informed on a topic, he or she must go to the scientific literature and read the original studies, and be able to interpret them. Even then, experts will disagree on the results and their meanings, but at least they have a common place from which to start their discussion.

The Scientific Method

To start the discussion of research design and interpretation, we must first think about the scientific method. The scientific method is fundamental in the design and interpretation of scientific information. We have all heard of the scientific method, but what is it? The scientific method consists of six basic steps. This is shown schematically in Figure 1–2, and described below:

1. Observe an occurrence—this can be something as simple as water flowing down hill, or something as complicated as the movement of muscle. Regardless, we observe something that interests us, but we do not know how it happens.

2. Make a hypothesis to explain our observation—a hypothesis can be little more than a guess, or it can be a well formulated idea, based on prior knowledge.

3. Make a prediction based on that hypothesis—here, you use the hypothesis about how things work to predict what might happen in another situation. We might predict that water will change direction if we tilt a pan a different way, or we might predict that by contracting a muscle we can make it lengthen in addition to shorten.

4. Design a study to test the predictions—in this step, you try to eliminate as many variables as possible, other than the one you are testing, so that you can say definitively that your prediction was correct or not. This is often a difficult part of the scientific method because, in real life, it is difficult to isolate only one variable. This is one of the aspects that make interpretation of studies difficult.

5. Compare the data collected to the prediction and conclude if the hypothesis was correct or incorrect. If the hypothesis was incorrect, then we modify the hypothesis to fit the results of the test—if the test didn't conform to your prediction, that can mean that the study was not done right, but it can also mean that the hypothesis was not correct, so what do you do? You can redesign the study to test the prediction in a better manner, and this is often done. If you are convinced that you did the study correctly, then you must change the hypothesis to fit the results of the study. This may mean that you have to completely "dump" the hypothesis, or it may mean that you only need to "tweak" it a little. This can be difficult scientifically and psychologically. Scientifically, you may not know, based on this experiment or your knowledge, how to modify your hypothesis, but it is also often hard for people to admit that their ideas were incorrect. Regardless, it is critical to good science that this step is taken.

6. Repeat steps 3–5 until you have shown that there are no other explanations for the observation. This may take a couple of attempts, but many scientists work for years developing and testing hypotheses, and this is the type of systematic approach that can yield a Nobel Prize for the truly pioneering scientists that gain this level of acclaim.

When reading scientific material, it is important to determine what hypothesis the researchers were testing. Most studies are conducted well and test a specific hypothesis, but some are not. The hypothesis is usually stated in the introduction of the report of the research, found in a scientific article. It may be as clearly stated as: "This study tested the hypothesis that water always flows downhill." Sometimes it is not stated that clearly, but you can determine the hypothesis from the questions posed in the introduction.

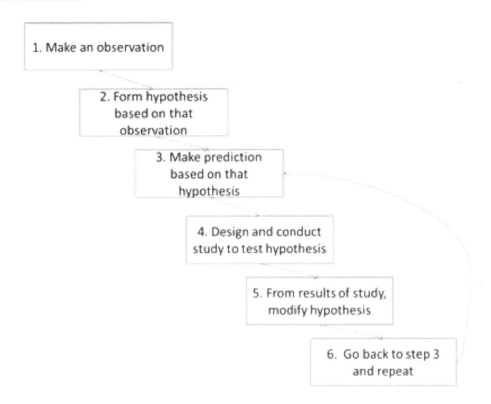

FIGURE 1–2. The steps involved in the scientific method.

Graph Reading

One of the simplest things to do when evaluating research is also one of the easiest to do improperly, and that is reading a graph. A graph is a picture of the relationship between two or more variables. These variables are classified as independent or dependent variables. The independent variable is the one that you think has an effect on other variables. Parameters such as age, gender, and fitness level are usually independent variables. The dependent variable is the one (or more) outcome(s) that you think are affected by the independent variable. Dependent variables include things such as the likelihood of developing heart disease, the heart rate during exercise, or the change in fitness level with a training program. Notice that we have included fitness level as both independent and dependent variables. This can be confusing, but if you think of the definition of independent and dependent variables, it does not need to be. If we evaluate the presence or absence of disease (dependent) in a population based on their fitness level, then fitness level is the independent variable. However, if we design different training programs to improve fitness, then the training program is the independent variable and the change in fitness is the dependent variable. In addition, there are extraneous variables. These are assumed to have no impact on the measurements being made, or are accounted for when the groups are randomized. Factors such as hair or eye color or the number of siblings one has are usually extraneous variables.

When graphing variables, the independent variable is placed on the horizontal or X axis, while the dependent variable is placed on the vertical or Y axis. For example, in the graph in Figure 1–3, body weight is the independent variable, and the amount of weight that can be lifted in a maximal bench press is the dependent variable. Can you see how bench press capability might be related to body weight?

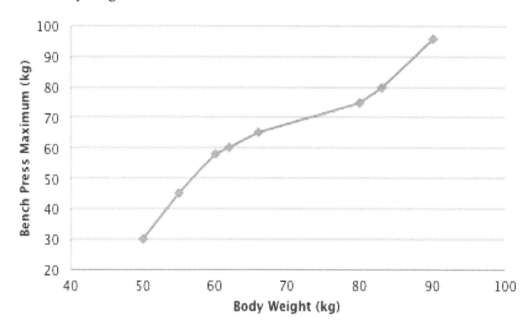

FIGURE 1–3. Graph of body weight vs. bench press capability. Which is the dependent and which is the independent variable?

It is important, when reading a graph, not to read too much into it. A graph such as Figure 1–3 shows a positive correlation between body weight and maximal bench press. That is, in general, as body weight increases, so does bench press capability. Does that mean that an increase in body weight *causes* an increase in bench press maximum? The answer is not necessarily. Large people are often stronger than smaller people because of more muscle mass, but if a small person became larger by addition of body fat, bench press maximum may not increase. There is a saying that "Correlation does not equal causality." This means that just because there is a correlation between two variables does not mean that one factor causes another. However, even though a correlation does not guarantee cause and effect, it is often a good starting point for future research. If you find a correlation between two variables, you can infer that they are related in some way and design future studies to examine that relationship.

A correlation can be positive or negative. The correlation in Figure 1–3 is positive. That is, as the independent variable increases, so does the dependent variable. There are also negative correlations, meaning that as one variable increases, the other decreases. This can be seen in Figure 1–4, where, as we age, our maximal heart rate decreases. Many students mistake the term negative correlation with a lack of a correlation, in which there is no relationship between the variables. Keep in mind that the two terms are not synonymous.

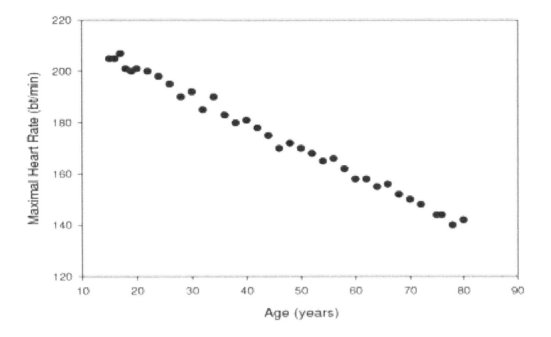

FIGURE 1-4. Age vs. maximal heart rate, an example of a negative correlation.

Study Designs

Another aspect of understanding how studies are conducted is understanding the distinctions between different types of study designs. Different hypotheses are best tested by different types of study design.

Study design, experimental

One of the most common study designs in exercise science is an experimental design. This type of study involves manipulating one or more independent variables to determine the effect that manipulation has on the dependent variable of interest. An example of an experimental study is the effect of a drug on blood pressure. To study the effects of drug X on blood pressure, we might divide our subject population into three groups. One group would get no drug, one a low dose of the drug, and one a high dose. Blood pressure would then be measured at the beginning of the experiment and after a duration thought to be sufficient for the drug to have an effect. This type of study design is used to help determine causality, as opposed to simply a correlation.

In an experimental design, there are number of ways by which the experimenter tries to eliminate extraneous variables or problems such as bias, where subjects know whether they have been given a treatment or not. In the example in the previous paragraph, one of the groups was not given the drug. This is referred to as the control group. Having a control group in a study is very important: it makes sure that the effect is not just because of the time taken for the experiment to be conducted or for natural changes. Many times, subjects have an idea about the effects of certain treatments. For that reason, a placebo is often used. A placebo is a treatment that looks or feels similar to the experimental treatment, but is known to have no effect. For example, if we divide the class into two groups and give one group a pill, but none to the other group, those who took the pill know they are the treatment group. But if we give the control group an inactive pill that looks and tastes like the pill given to the treatment group, the groups do not know whether they have been given the treatment or not.

Another method to help eliminate bias in a study is called blinding. Blinding means not revealing to the subjects which treatment they have been given—the control or an experimental level. This is referred to as single blind. There may also be bias among researchers. Scientists are people just like all of us. They have opinions about what should happen, and sometimes those biases creep in to the research. For that reason, there are also what are termed double blind experiments. In this case, neither the subject nor the researcher knows which subject has been given which treatment. In a double blind experiment, a collaborator or assistant will give out the treatments so that the researcher conducting the experiment doesn't know. A double blind experiment is generally considered a very strong design and we try to use this whenever possible.

Study design, observational

In an observational study design, direct manipulation of the independent variables is not done. Instead, subjects are often grouped by the independent variable. For example, many studies evaluate the difference in response by age, by gender, or by fitness level. There are three primary types of observational study: cross-sectional, retrospective, and prospective.

There are two types of cross-sectional study. In one, people are selected from a population and both the independent and dependent variables are measured in all subjects at one time. This allows a correlation to be made between the variables. For example, the independent variable might be fitness level and the dependent variable may be an indicator of heart disease. The level of fitness would be compared to the number or severity of heart disease indicators. In the other type of cross-sectional study, subjects are still chosen from a population, but are divided into two or more groups. These groups may be age, gender, or fitness level. Again, the dependent and independent variables are measured, but instead of evaluating the correlation between the variables, comparisons are made between the means of the groups. In either case, this does not allow us to evaluate the cause of the association, only that there is an association (correlation) between the variables, or that there are differences in the dependent variable between the groups.

A retrospective study is also called a case-control study design. In a retrospective study, different levels of the dependent variable are used and the independent variable is measured retrospectively. For example, a researcher can look at a population, divide them into people with and without heart disease, then go back and evaluate their physical activity level for the previous ten years. Again, this type of study does not allow the establishment of cause, only of correlations. It is also subject to errors and biases in that people either may not remember their level of activity or the food they ate, or may not be as willing to admit to being inactive or having fried butter at the state fair.

A prospective study evaluates people over time for both the independent and dependent variables. We might examine the muscle strength of people who do and do not use resistance training as they age from thirty to sixty years, a period when strength declines generally occur, but may be delayed by training. This type of study is also sometimes referred to as a longitudinal study.

In addition to these specific types of studies, combinations of these can be made. For example, we can employ an experimental approach in a longitudinal fashion if we start out with two groups of people and treat them the same, but train one for many years and not the other. These designs, though, are somewhat complicated and the subject of a more advanced course.

Reading the Scientific Literature

Key to the study of science in any field is the ability to evaluate the scientific literature. You now know something about study design and the scientific method, which should allow you to evaluate some of the articles that appear in science journals. It is critically important to get information from original sources as often as possible. While popular magazines may be a good source for what is currently being done in the fitness field, with information on new diets, supplements, or training programs, they are not the best places to find accurate information. While some popular articles are balanced and provide a lot of good information, in some cases, the authors of the articles are attempting to promote a specific point of view and do not provide a balanced approach to the article. In other cases, they do not have the knowledge to determine what is correct and what is not, so are unable to provide a balanced approach.

Not even all scientific articles, though are without errors or biases, but because of the process of getting them published, most of the errors and opinions are removed. This is because of a process referred to as peer review. When a scientific article is submitted to a journal editor for publication, it is usually sent to two to three experts in the field for review. These experts read the article, evaluate it for scientific merit, accuracy, and bias, and make suggestions for revisions. Only after the revisions have been made and the articles accepted by the reviewers and the editor are they published. Therefore, articles taken from scientific journals are usually considered to be the best sources for accurate, up-to-date information.

Scientific articles come in two main types. There are research papers and review articles. Research papers are reports of one or more closely-related experiments. They are divided into different sections. The introduction describes the background and need for the study so that the reader learns about studies that have preceded this one and any disagreements between previous studies that lead to the need for the current one. It usually contains a statement of the hypothesis, or at least the questions that are to be answered. The methods section describes, in detail, the manner in which the study was conducted. It will usually describe any tests performed, the order of the tests, the types of subjects involved and how they were selected, and the method by which the data that was collected was analyzed. The results section gives a detailed description of the data collected, the results of any statistical analyses, and usually has graphs and tables that help describe the data that was collected. This section does not usually interpret that data except to say whether or not there were any correlations or whether or not different results were statistically meaningful (significant). In the discussion section, data interpretation takes place. This section is devoted to describing how the data supported or refuted the hypothesis. It is also the section where the data from the current study is compared to that collected by others, whether it agrees or disagrees and why, and how it adds to the knowledge base on the topic.

The other primary type of scientific article is the review article. This type of article is usually written to summarize the current knowledge in a particular topic. For example, one might write a review article on the effect of exercise on heart disease. In this review, the author(s) will assemble a large number of references and try to present a balanced picture of the knowledge in the area and controversies that exist. They do not describe individual experiments except to try to discern strengths and weaknesses in the knowledge in the area. In short, a review article is similar in nature to term papers that you might write for an assignment in a class, but usually in considerably more depth. While the authors, reviewers, and editors try to prevent too much of a person's opinions and biases from coming in to a review article, it is still the author(s) interpretation of work done by themselves and others, so a review article is at least one step away from the research papers described above, and subject to some potential bias.

Some people refer to the scientific papers as primary sources and the review articles as secondary sources, and this is a good description. A primary source is the best place to get the most accurate information about a topic, without relying on the interpretations of others about the data. The secondary sources, though, are not without usefulness. If a review article is written by a person considered a true expert in the field, it can give the reader a very good idea of what is known, what is not known about a topic, and what is suspected without having to find many scientific articles on that area. It is a good way to find out information on something on which you are not an expert, but need to learn about.

Glossary

Blinding—a method of experimentation in which the subject (single blind) or both the subject and the investigator (double blind) does not know who has been administered the experimental manipulation.

Control—a group within a study that has not been administered the variable of interest.

Cross-sectional Study—a method of experiment in which different groups are evaluated for the independent and dependent variable at one time.

Dependent variable—a variable that is affected by other variables.

Hypothesis—part of the scientific method that involves explaining an observation that has been seen.

Independent variable—a variable that has (or is thought to have) an effect on other variables.

Placebo—a treatment that looks and feels like the treatment in order to mask the control from the experimental group.

Prospective Study—a type of scientific study in which subjects are evaluated for both the dependent and independent variables over time.

Retrospective Study—a method of scientific study in which different levels of a dependent variables are used and the independent variable is then measured.

General References

Housh, T. J., D. J. Housh and G. O. Johnson (eds). 2008. *Introduction to Exercise Science*, 3rd ed. Scottsdale, AZ: Holcomb Hathaway Publishers.

Potteiger, J. A. 2011. *ACSM's Introduction to Exercise Science*. Philadelphia: Lippincott Williams and Wilkins Publishers.

Shea, C. H. and D. L. Wright. 1997. *An Introduction to Human Movement*. Boston: Allyn and Bacon Publishers.

Tipton, C. M. (ed). 2006. *ACSM's Advanced Exercise Physiology*. Philadelphia: Lippincott Williams and Wilkins Publishers.

Chapter 2

HOMEOSTASIS, BIOENERGETICS, AND SKELETAL MUSCLE PHYSIOLOGY

P hysiology is a central thread in exercise science, as well as most biomedical science. Physiology features prominently in most exercise science, kinesiology, and movement science degrees, as well as in athletic training, and essentially all medical curricula. Most colleges and universities offer basic classes in anatomy and physiology, as well as advanced courses in human, animal, comparative, and/or exercise physiology. In addition, exercise physiology programs typically offer clinically-oriented physiology classes like Exercise Testing and Prescription. The study of physiology is often broken down by organ system, for example, cardiovascular physiology, renal (kidney) physiology, and muscle physiology. We will focus on the systems that are most directly involved in exercise—muscle, heart, and lungs. Before we get to those systems, however, we will study the most fundamental concept in physiology, homeostasis.

Part 1. Homeostasis

The cornerstone of physiology is a concept called homeostasis. Homeostasis is a paradigm (what does that word mean?) for how living systems respond to stresses, like exercise, or heat, or high altitude. The word itself is Greek, from two roots—homeo, meaning "similar" and stasis, meaning "stoppage." Similar-stoppage isn't a particularly enlightening translation, but if we translate less literally, the term refers to holding something the same—preventing change. Still, in order to understand the concept of homeostasis, we need to go back to its origin—before the term "homeostasis" itself existed.

Claude Bernard and Walter Cannon

The French physiologist Claude Bernard, working in the mid-1800's, noted that the conditions inside an animal's body were not a simple reflection of the conditions outside the animal. Specifically, living things (Bernard would have specified warm blooded vertebrates) set up an internal environment that is more hospitable to their cells than the outside environment would be. For example, the temperature inside your body stays around 37°C irrespective of whether it's -4°C outside or 40°C outside. Bernard further noted that setting up and maintaining the internal environment required constant vigilance. He said that all of the animal's "vital mechanisms" (organs and functions) were dedicated to the task of protecting and preserving the internal environment.

Claude Bernard's work was translated into English and republished in 1927. Around that time, an American physiologist, Walter Cannon, was also thinking about the consistency of the internal environment. Cannon was well aware of Bernard's work and conducted his own with a similar perspective. Cannon contrived the term "homeostasis" to describe the compensatory processes by which the body functioned to limit variations in the internal environment. Both the word and the concept of homeostasis became much more broadly appreciated with the publication of Cannon's 1932 book *The Wisdom of the Body*. This book was coffee table reading, at least for the educated elite.

Cannon was also interested in *how* homeostasis is achieved—the mechanisms. In this regard, he focused his attention on the branch of the nervous system that we now call the autonomic nervous system (more on that later). Hormones had only recently been discovered when *The Wisdom of the Body* was published, but Cannon and others quickly recognized their relevance to homeostasis.

At this point, let's stop for a moment and consider what aspects of the internal environment are homeostatically regulated. One has already been cited—body temperature. Other homeostatically regulated parameters include blood pressure, blood glucose (sugar) concentration, and blood gas (oxygen, carbon dioxide) concentrations. Many homeostatic parameters are commonly measured in a doctor's office or with routine blood tests. That should make sense—homeostasis is related to health. You might think that values like heart rate and respiratory rate are also homeostatically regulated, but they are not. Rather, heart rate, respiratory rate, as well as blood hormone concentrations, are mechanisms to control other, critical functions. For example, respiratory rate itself isn't particularly important. However, blood oxygen content is very important, and alterations in respiratory rate can impact oxygenation.

Assignment 2–1.　　How many homeostatically regulated body parameters not listed above can you list?

Homeostatic Regulation and the Negative Feedback Loop

Cannon emphasized that homeostasis is a *dynamic* process and that regulated parameters are not truly constant but actually fluctuate up and down around an average value or "set point" value. For example, while your average body temperature is around 37°C, you might be a bit lower in the morning, perhaps 36.5°C, and a bit higher after lunch, perhaps 37.5°C. Other controlled variables may fluctuate around their set points on a shorter time scale—minutes or seconds. Cannon reasoned that these fluctuations were not the sign of a faulty system, but rather the consequence of an ever changing system. In medicine, it can be a challenge to identify when an "abnormal" value of a controlled variable actually reflects a problem, versus when it is within tolerable limits for a particular person in a particular condition. For example, think about your arterial (blood) oxygen pressure. Do you think that healthy college students in Mexico City, Mexico or

Quito, Ecuador (both over 2000 m/ 7,000 ft. elevation) have the same arterial oxygen pressure as do healthy college students in Boston or Miami (both at approximately sea level)?

The oscillation in homeostatically regulated parameters is also related to the primary method by which they are controlled. Most homeostatically regulated variables are controlled by a mechanism known as **negative feedback regulation**, or a **negative feedback loop**. Negative feedback regulation is an old engineering principle, and the application of this concept to biological systems was the result of engineers collaborating with physiologists.

The negative feedback loop has physical, tangible components and conceptual, intangible components. The tangible ones will be described first. Every negative feedback loop has the following parts:

Sensor—this is the part of the body that can sense or detect the regulated variable.

Integrator—this is the part of the body that can interpret information coming from the sensor, and send messages out to the effector. In the body, the integrator is the brain.

Effector—this is the part of the body that can affect or change the regulated variable.

The sensor, integrator, and effector are real, identifiable parts of the body. The intangible components; set point, threshold, and error signal, are more easily understood by example. We'll use first a non-biological example of negative feedback regulation—the home heating/cooling system. As you know, most homes have a thermostat. You can decide what temperature you want the room temperature to be, and set the thermostat accordingly. In order for the indoor temperature to be maintained at your chosen temperature, let's say 20°C (68°F), there has to be something in the thermostat that can SENSE the actual temperature inside the residence. An example of a temperature sensor is a thermometer. That temperature information must be sent to an INTEGRATOR, and these days, that's a computer chip inside the thermostat. The integrator has to decide what, if any, action is needed to achieve the desired temperature of 20°C. For example, in winter, the indoor temperature will tend to drop, until it is equal with the outdoor temperature, which might be around 0°C (32°F). In order to keep the temperature at 20°C, the integrator must tell the furnace to come on. The furnace is the EFFECTOR because it can change the temperature. On the other hand, if it's summer, the outdoor temperature may be hotter than the desired indoor temperature. In that case, the integrator needs to tell the air conditioning unit to operate. The temperature you select and dial into the thermostat is a conceptual parameter called the SET POINT. This is the temperature you want to maintain. Note, there will be some variation around this temperature. If your set point is 20°C, do you expect the heater to click on if the temperature drops to 19.8°C? How about if it's 19.6°C? 19°C? The point is, there is some THRESHOLD for action. The integrator has to decide when the deviation between the desired (set point) temperature and the actual temperature is too big to tolerate. That's when it tells the effector to make a change. The deviation between the actual value of a variable and the set point value is called the ERROR SIGNAL—that's the negative feedback in this loop.

All of this reasoning applies to biological systems as well. The set point temperature in your body is around 37°C. If you are standing outside in January, you may need to take action in order to defend that internal temperature against the cold external temperature. For example, you could follow your mother's advice and put a coat on! (That's called behavioral thermoregulation.) What are some of the possible *physiological* actions that can help you keep warm? Likewise, if it's summer in Phoenix, Arizona, you will likely have to defend your internal temperature, in this case against external temperatures over 40°C. What are your effectors in that case?

TABLE 2–1. Components of a negative feedback loop.

Physical:	Conceptual:
Sensor	Error Signal
Integrator	Set Point
Effector	Threshold

Assignment 2–2.   Be prepared to illustrate (draw) a negative feedback loop for the regulation of a homeostatically controlled variable.

Homeostasis and Exercise

Perhaps you've been wondering, what does this have to do with exercise? Exercise stresses the body, and without compensation, would tend to change the internal environment. Among other challenges, exercise increases the rates of nutrient and oxygen use, increases waste production, and increases heat production. All of these challenges could alter the value of a homeostatically regulated parameter, for example, the heat produced during exercise can raise body temperature. Consequently, heat must be dissipated in order to keep body temperature within acceptable limits. Sweating is an active mechanism for increasing evaporative heat loss. What other regulated parameters are potentially altered by exercise? What are the body's compensations?

Exercise is just one possible stress on the body—there are more. A stressor is any condition or process that has the potential to push a controlled variable beyond the acceptable range of values. What other potential stresses can you think of? What aspect(s) of your local environment pose particular stresses on homeostasis?

Assignment 2–3.   List three potential stresses to homeostatic regulation of the internal environment. Be specific. For each stressor, indicate which homeostatically regulated variable is affected and if it is likely to be increased or decreased.

The Homeostatic Continuum

We're going to return to the notion that homeostasis describes a dynamic process, and thereby refine our understanding of set points. Dr. Donald Jackson, Professor Emeritus at Brown University, studied homeostatic processes in animals from dogs to turtles. In a 1987 paper he discussed the continuum of homeostasis:

> *"Homeostasis is not a single optimal control condition but rather a variety or continuum that varies with the animal's circumstances."*
>
> (Jackson, 1987)

In order to understand what Dr. Jackson had in mind, consider animals that hibernate, like groundhogs or bears. During the late spring, summer, and fall, groundhogs have an internal temperature, as well as other internal parameters, that are similar to yours. However, during the winter (i.e., during hibernation), a groundhog's body temperature is held at about 8°C, and many other internal parameters are very *unlike* yours. Is this a homeostatic break down, or does it make sense? There's little food for a groundhog in winter, and maintaining a high body temperature when the outside temperature is low costs a lot of energy. Lowering body temperature saves energy just like lowering the temperature on a residential thermostat. The groundhog's strategy involves two distinct conditions and the set points differ greatly between them. Dr. Jackson continued:

> *". . . set points or regulated values are not fixed, but may . . . change depending on ambient conditions or because of changing physiological conditions or demands."*
>
> (Jackson, 1987)

Can you think of any changes in ambient conditions or physiological demands that cause set points to change in humans? Consider high altitude—are any homeostatically regulated parameters different at high altitude compared to sea level? What important, but temporary, physiological condition can affect only *half* of the population and involves a lot of set point changes?

Assignment 2–4.   Write down at least one example of a regulated change in the set point of a homeostatically regulated parameter in a human. Describe the condition, the affected parameter, and the direction (increase or decrease) of the change.

Homeostasis versus Steady-State

We'll close this section with a note on terminology. It's important not to confuse the terms *homeostasis* and *steady-state*. This entire section has been focused on homeostasis. That term describes the dynamic process whereby the value (set point) of a parameter is defended against changes. Homeostasis is active. Steady-state has a simpler meaning. Steady-state means that a parameter is constant over some period of time. That parameter may or may not be homeostatically regulated. For example, respiratory (breathing) rate is not homeostatically regulated. However, it can be steady-state. If your respiratory rate is 20 breaths per minute now, and stays at that value for the next five minutes, then your respiratory rate was steady-state for those five minutes. Consider the (made up) example on the next page that contrasts homeostatic regulation of body temperature with body temperature at steady state.

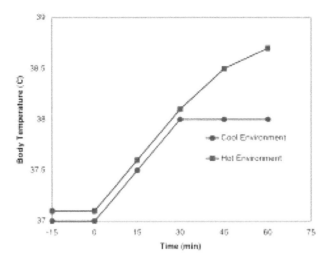

FIGURE 2–1. Body temperature before exercise and during 60 minutes of jogging exercise in a cool environment (blue circles) and a hot environment (red squares). Data are made up for this example.

Assignment 2–5.   Using Figure 2–1, write down: (a) the time periods over which body temperature is steady-state, in each environment (cool, hot) and (b) the time periods over which body temperature is homeo-statically regulated, in each environment. Come to class prepared to justify your answers.

Part 2. Bioenergetics

Irrefutably, living requires energy. In this section on bioenergetics, we will consider how animals use the energy in foods to power the activities of living, in particular, exercise. Of course, we will not have time to go into great detail—you can expand your knowledge of bioenergetics in classes such as Anatomy and Physiology, Exercise Physiology, and Biochemistry.

Energy

In science, you will read about different "types" of energy, depending on the context. Particularly in physics and engineering classes, you may see terms such as kinetic energy, potential energy, heat, and work. In reality, these terms all describe the same thing, and we know this because they are all measured in the same units. The system international (SI) unit for energy is the joule (J). You will also see energy measured in calories, or on food labels in Calories (1000 calories = 1 Calorie). How many joules are in a calorie? (Look it up.) In engineering, you may also see energy measured as British Thermal Units (BTU). In physics, you may encounter energy described in units of electron volts (eV). One electron volt is a tiny, tiny fraction of a joule (electrons are really small!). All these different units are analogous to the different units we have for measuring distance, for example meters (or kilometers), feet, yards, miles, furlongs, etc. The distance from Dallas to Houston doesn't depend on the measurement unit—it's 226 miles or 364 km. Likewise, the energy in a typical apple is about 100 Calories, or 419 kilojoules, or 397 BTU, or 2.61×10^{24} eV.

But what about heat and work? Do not confuse heat with temperature. Temperature is measured in degrees Celsius, or Fahrenheit, or Kelvin. To raise the temperature of something, we have to put in energy, or in other words, we have to HEAT it. Likewise, work is a description of how much energy it takes to accomplish something, and it's measured in joules. For example, we could calculate the amount of work (energy) required to carry a pumpkin to the top of the Empire State building in New York. Why does it require more work to take a pumpkin to the top than to take a paper clip to the top?

The first law of thermodynamics assures us that energy can be transformed from one 'form' to another, for example, from work to heat. That's a good thing, because living things need to make energy transformations. Food contains stored potential energy that animals need to use for all bodily functions (growth, movement, etc.). In order to exploit the energy in food, animals must first put that energy into a usable "currency." An analogy may be helpful here. In our economy, we get things we need and want by using currency, or money. To get money, we work. It doesn't matter what kind of work you do—fighting fires, interpreting law, repairing sinks, or teaching—in all cases we are paid in dollars (money). We want dollars because we can use them to pay rent, buy groceries, or bid on eBay. Likewise, the foods we eat are varied, but there is only one energy "currency" in the body, a molecule known as ATP (adenosine triphosphate). ATP can be "spent" to do all the energy-requiring processes in the body—growth, repair, locomotion, reproduction, etc.

ATP

ATP was discovered by Karl Lohmann in 1929 (Nobelprize.org). Over the next decade or so, the role of ATP in muscle contraction was elucidated. Determining the ways in which cells synthesize ATP was a challenge, and the 1997 Nobel Prize in Chemistry was awarded to three scientists in part for their work on how cells generate ATP. ATP is a molecule that has three basic parts. One part is the adenine, a molecule made up of carbon, hydrogen, and nitrogen atoms. The second part is a sugar molecule, ribose, which you will see again when you study DNA. The third part is a trio of phosphate groups—it's called TRIphosphate because there are three. Phosphates contain a phosphorus atom (P in the periodic table) as well as oxygen atoms. The three phosphates are linked in a chain attached to the ribose. If you take the third phosphate off ATP, it becomes ADP (adenosine DIphosphate). If you take the third and second phosphates off, you are left with AMP (adenosine MONOphosphate). Breaking off (or "cleaving") the third phosphate from the second (ATP to ADP) releases about 30 KJ per mole. [A mole is a quantity—6.02×10^{23}. This is analogous to a dozen—"dozen" is the word for 12, "mole" is the word for 6.02×10^{23}.] The energy released when ATP is broken down into ADP is used to power bodily functions, including muscle contractions.

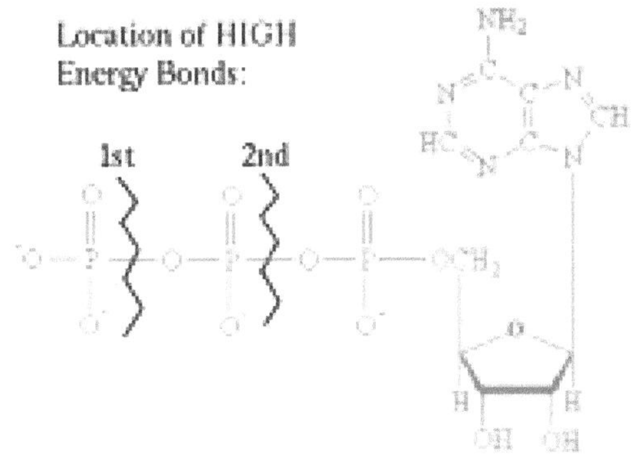

FIGURE 2–2. ATP. Blue–phosphates; pink–ribose; red–adenine.

The body stores very little ATP—there's no equivalent to a savings account. So, in order to keep spending ATP, the body needs to constantly make ATP. To do this, cells must take the energy found in the varied chemical bonds of food and convert it into energy stored in ATP. Obviously, part of that process is digestion. We're not going to cover digestion. What we will discuss generally falls under the rubric of metabolism or bioenergetics. So, we'll pick up from the point where the body has put fundamental energy sources (carbohydrate, fat, protein) into cells.

Energy Sources

The macronutrients, carbohydrate, fat, and protein, will be covered in depth in Chapter 7, Fitness and Wellness. For now, we'll just cover the basics so everyone is comfortable with the terms.

Carbohydrates are made of carbon, hydrogen, and oxygen. Sugars are carbohydrates. The simplest sugar is a monosaccharide—mono for one, saccharide for sugar. Glucose is a monosaccharide. The stuff that comes in sugar packets is sucrose, a disaccharide. Sucrose is the combination of glucose and fructose. Lactose, the sugar in milk (which some people cannot digest = lactose intolerant), is also a disaccharide. The term for three or more sugars is polysaccharide. Plants store carbohydrates as a polysaccharide called starch. Animals store carbohydrates as a polysaccharide called glycogen. There are other polysaccharides, such as cellulose (a "fiber"). Vertebrate animals including humans can digest starch and glycogen, but lack the enzymes necessary to digest fiber. Nonetheless, lots of mammals from rabbits to cows to elephants live on high fiber plants such as grasses. In other words, they do get energy from fiber. How is that accomplished?

Assignment 2–6. The energy yield from carbohydrates is about 4 Calories/gram (4000 cal/gram or 17000 J/gram or 17 KJ/gram). An "average" 70 kg man has about 10 g of glucose in the blood, or about 40 Calories. He has an additional 60 g of glycogen stored in the liver and 350 g of glycogen stored in skeletal muscles (across many muscles—not all in the biceps!). How many Calories (or cal or joules) does this "average" man have stored in his body? (I've listed all stores.) How many days worth of energy is that?

The second fundamental energy source is fat. Fat is made of carbon and hydrogen atoms. It comes in several forms, but most relevant to energy metabolism are triglycerides and fatty acids. Fatty acids are long chains of carbon and hydrogen. Below is an example of a fatty acid.

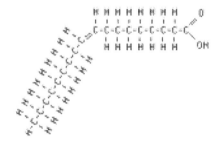

Oleic acid, a monounsaturated fatty acid.
Note that the double bond is *cis*; this is
the common natural configuration.

FIGURE 2-3. Oleic Acid—$C_{18}H_{34}O_2$, an example of a fatty acid.

Saturated fatty acids have no double bonds between carbons and all carbons (except the last one bound to oxygen) are bound to at least two hydrogen atoms. In contrast, unsaturated fatty acids, such as oleic acid, have one or more double bonds between two carbons. Oleic acid is mono-unsaturated because there is only one double bond. Polyunsaturated fatty acids have at least two double bonds. Fatty acids can be found in the blood and in cells, but are not the storage form of fat. The storage form for both plants and animals is triglyceride, the linkage of three (TRI) fatty acids to a single glycerol molecule. A "normal" 70 kg man has about 14 kg of triglyceride stored in adipocytes (fat cells) and another 0.5 kg of fat stored across the skeletal muscles. Fat has an energy content of 9 Calories/gram (38 KJ/gram), so this person has over 130,000 Calories of energy stored in fat. How many days' worth is that?

Protein is also a potential energy source. Protein is different from carbohydrate and fat in that in addition to carbon, hydrogen, and oxygen, protein also contains nitrogen. In order for protein to be used as energy, the nitrogen must be removed, a process called deamination. The basic units of proteins are molecules called amino acids. Examples of amino acids include alanine, leucine, and valine. You can easily find a list of the 20 biologically common amino acids in books or online. Protein can provide about 4 Calories/gram (17 KJ/gram) but protein is not the preferred energy source for humans. Under normal circumstances, less than 5% of the energy a person uses comes from protein. The percentage can be increased by starvation, prolonged exercise (like a triathlon), or a low carbohydrate diet such as Atkins. The protein in your body is either structural or functional. Enzymes are proteins that catalyze (~facilitate) chemical reactions inside living things. Antibodies are proteins involved in immunity. Your muscles have a large protein content, and even your bones have protein in them.

Carbohydrate, fat, and protein are the fundamental energy sources, but as mentioned previously, the energy contained within them must be transferred to ATP before the energy can be "spent." Next, we're going to cover three pathways by which muscle cells (in particular) can generate ATP.

ATP Generation in Muscle Cells

The fastest way a muscle cell can produce ATP is to break down a molecule called creatine phosphate. Creatine itself can be obtained in the diet from meat, and in addition it can be synthesized in the body from amino acids. When a phosphate group (as seen in ATP) is attached to the creatine via a "high energy" phosphate bond, it becomes creatine phosphate (CP) or phosphocreatine (PC). Muscle cells store CP—there's about 5–6 times more CP than ATP in a muscle cell. One CP can be broken to make *one* ATP. The energy in the creatine to phosphate bond is released and used to put a phosphate group on ADP to make ATP. This process is fast but limited by the finite supply of CP. Muscles have enough CP to power perhaps 10 or 20 sec of maximal intensity exercise. Ten to twenty seconds is not enough time for most activities, so obviously, other mechanisms of ATP generation are needed.

Assignment 2–7.   Creatine is sold legally as an ergogenic aid (an exercise/work enhancer). What types of exercise would you predict creatine to affect? What types of exercise do you think would not be affected by creatine supplementation? What evidence supports a positive ergogenic effect of creatine supplementation? (Where would you find good quality evidence?)

As mentioned previously, carbohydrate is an important energy source. Most cells, including muscle cells, can break down (or lyse) glucose or glycogen (stored glucose) to make ATP in a process known as glycolysis. Glycolysis has many steps. Inside living systems, energy release must be done via a series of small reactions. Enzymes catalyze (facilitate) each of these small reactions. By comparison, the energy (caloric) content of food is determined using a device called a bomb calorimeter. Do you think a bomb calorimeter uses a series of small reactions?

In order to make ATP using the energy in glucose, two ATP must be invested in the early stages of glycolysis. Eventually, the six carbon glucose molecule is broken into two, three carbon molecules and ultimately, four ATP are made. The net ATP production is only two, because four minus the two invested is two. The three carbon end product of glycolysis is called pyruvic acid.

$$C_6H_{12}O_6 + 2NAD^+ \rightarrow 2C_3H_4O_3 + 2NADHH^+ \text{ w/ 2ATP formed}$$

Pyruvic acid has two potential fates. It can be converted to lactic acid or, with the loss of another carbon, it can be converted into a molecule called acetyl-CoA and used to make more ATP. Before we talk about that second process, we'll focus on the conversion of pyruvic acid into lactic acid.

$$C_3H_4O_3 + NADHH^+ \rightarrow C_3H_6O_3 + NAD^+$$
$$\text{Pyruvic acid} \qquad\qquad \text{Lactic acid}$$

This conversion is catalyzed by an enzyme called lactate dehydrogenase. Advantages of this conversion include that it is relatively fast and "regenerates" NAD+, which is needed for further break down of glucose to make more ATP (note the NAD+ in the glucose reaction above). A disadvantage is that lactic acid is an acid, i.e., it has the potential to affect pH. In water, most of the lactic acid will lose an H+ ion and become lactate, while at the same time, the cell will become more acidic due to the increased concentration of H+ ion. The cell will release some of the lactate and H+ ions into the blood, so the blood will also become more acidic over time. The temporary acidification isn't necessarily a big problem, but it must be accommodated—there are buffers in the blood that protect against big changes in pH.

What happens to the lactate itself? There are three possible fates for lactate. Although it's a debatable point, it's probable that some of it is transported into the mitochondria of the cell and used there as an aerobic energy source (see section on aerobic ATP production, on the next page). More confidently, we know that lactate is also released from cells, into the blood. The heart, other muscles, the kidney, and the liver can take up lactate and use it as a fuel source. A significant amount of the energy in glucose is still contained within lactate. Additionally, the liver can take up lactate and convert it back to glucose via a process known as gluconeogenesis. Only the liver can do this—other organs lack the necessary enzymes. As a general rule of thumb, about three quarters of the lactate produced during submaximal exercise is taken up by various tissues and consumed for energy while about a quarter is converted back to glucose by the liver.

Lactate is at the center of several popular myths. The most common incorrect statement about lactic acid is that it is responsible for muscle soreness. Experiments in which lactic acid was infused have shown this isn't the case. Any acid can produce an acute sense of pain, but lactic acid *per se* isn't the main culprit in either immediate or delayed muscle soreness from exercise. There may not be one single cause of muscle soreness, but there are many candidates including prostaglandins, bradykinin, and substance P.

Aerobic ATP Production

Aerobic means with oxygen. We all know that animals—from invertebrates to mammals—require oxygen. Oxygen is needed for efficient production of ATP. Aerobic phosphorylation—the process of sticking a third phosphate group onto ADP—takes place within subcellular structures known as mitochondria. Aerobic ATP production inside the mitochondria involves the interaction of the Krebs or Citric Acid Cycle and the electron transport chain. The Krebs Cycle yields carbon dioxide and electrons. The electron transport chain uses oxygen and produces water and the potential energy needed to make ATP.

Oxidation-Reduction Reactions

Before we continue, we need to make a digression to oxidation-reduction reactions. For success in both physiology and chemistry, it's essential you understand oxidation and reduction—the loss and gain of electrons. There are several pneumonics for remembering these two reactions, for example OIL RIG (oxidation is loss, reduction is gain). A nicer way of saying that an atom or molecule loses electrons is to say it "donates" electrons. Likewise, the atom or molecule that becomes reduced "accepts" electrons. When a molecule is reduced, its charge will also be reduced (by the addition of negative electrons). Electrons travel in pairs—it's rare to have an unaccompanied electron (and when there is one, it's usually dangerous). Oxygen is "desirous" of two electrons. (Obviously an atom can't be desirous, but it's easier to remember this way.) Oxygen wants two electrons due to its electron configuration and a principle known as the octet rule. The octet rule says that atoms behave in a manner that increases the chances of getting eight electrons in the outer, or valance, shell. Oxygen has eight electrons total (eight electrons match its eight protons), however only six of those electrons are in the #2 (valance) shell. The configuration is 1s2, 2s2, 2p4. Oxygen "desires" two more electrons to bring the 2p total to its capacity of six, and the valance shell total to eight—2s2, 2p6, thereby satisfying the octet rule. You'll likely hear much more about electron configuration in chemistry classes.

The upshot of the octet rule is that oxygen will readily accept two electrons, and in so doing, become reduced. The electron donor becomes oxidized (this is why oxygen is known as an oxidizing agent). What's oxidized iron called?

Assignment 2–8. What element has the electron configuration 1s2, 2s2, 2p6? How many protons does it have? (That second question is a hint.) How many electrons does it need to follow the octet rule? What other element(s) would you predict "want" two electrons, like oxygen? What element(s) would you predict readily give up two electrons (become oxidized)?

Aerobic ATP Production, Continued

You will recall that anaerobic glycolysis results in the production of two pyruvic acid molecules from one glucose molecule. The pyruvic acid can be anaerobically converted to lactic acid. That's fast, but not energy efficient. To extract more energy out of the glucose, the pyruvic acid must be further broken down inside a mitochondrion. The first step is the removal of another carbon (with production of CO_2) and the addition of something called coenzyme A to produce acetyl-CoA. Acetyl-CoA is then combined with a four carbon molecule and taken through a series of steps that ultimately converts the two remaining carbons from the original glucose into carbon dioxide (while regenerating the original four carbon molecule—so it's a cycle). Hans Krebs and Fritz Lipmann shared the Nobel Prize in 1953 for discovery and description of the Citric Acid (Krebs) Cycle and coenzyme A (http://www.jbc.org/content/280/21/e18.full).

The other process occurring in the Krebs Cycle is the removal of hydrogen atoms (pairs of protons and electrons) that were once associated with the glucose molecule. The electrons reduce NAD+ to NADHH+ and FAD to FADH2. The NADHH+ and FADH2 take the electrons to the electron transport chain, which is a series of molecules embedded in the inner mitochondrial membrane. The electron transport chain is like a bucket brigade—one molecule receives a pair of electrons, becomes reduced, but then gives them up to the next molecule, and in so doing is re-oxidized. At the very end of this chain waits oxygen. Oxygen will receive two electrons and keep them. In the process, oxygen also inherits the two protons that originally came with the electrons. Two electrons plus two protons equals two hydrogen atoms. One oxygen plus two hydrogen atoms makes $O + H + H = H_2O$ or WATER.

The electron transport chain is like a downhill cascade of electrons. In this sense, it is analogous to the downhill flow of water. When water flows downhill, energy is released. When the electrons flow "downhill," the energy released is indirectly used to add a phosphate group to ADP to make ATP. Roughly, each pair of electrons releases enough energy to make three ATP.

So far, we've only discussed the metabolism of glucose. Fat and protein can also be converted to acetyl-CoA. In the case of fat, the fatty acids are chopped into two carbon units via a process known as beta-oxidation. Protein must be broken down into the component amino acids, which conveniently include two carbons. As mentioned previously, the nitrogen in protein must be removed for the conversion to acetyl-coA. It is important to note that neither fat nor protein can be used anaerobically. Only carbohydrate can be used anaerobically, but all three energy sources can be used aerobically inside mitochondria.

Assignment 2–9.   In the famous James Bond books and movies, the agents were issued sodium cyanide pills in case they were captured by the enemy. Sadly, in real life, seven people died in 1982 from taking Tylenol capsules that had been laced with potassium cyanide. Cyanide poisoning inhibits the aerobic production of ATP. What step in the process is affected?

Efficiency and Combination of Aerobic and Anaerobic Pathways

Just as not all the energy in gasoline is captured in a car engine, you don't capture all the energy in food when you make ATP. Much of the energy is released as heat (as in a car). If you combust glucose, it will release 686 kcal/mole. Aerobic metabolism of one molecule of glucose yields about 32 ATP (number will vary slightly, depending on the accounting). When you use the ATP (break it down into ADP and inorganic phosphate), you get about 7.3 kcal/mole. With a little basic math, these numbers indicate an efficiency of about 34%. If glucose is used anaerobically (resulting in two molecules of lactate), only two ATP are made. That efficiency is really poor—only about 2%! But, there are times when we need rapid ATP production and in addition, there are some cells, such as red blood cells, which lack mitochondria. Therefore, there will always be some degree of anaerobic metabolism. Generally, at rest, most ATP production is aerobic. As exercise intensity increases, a greater and greater contribution of anaerobic metabolism is seen. Thus, for very high intensity activities, like 100 m sprinting, shot put, etc., 90+% of the ATP may come from a combination of CP breakdown and anaerobic carbohydrate use. The opposite is true for lower intensity, longer duration exercise—for 10 km running (for example), over 90% of the ATP comes from aerobic metabolism. As a general rule of thumb, the 50/50 point is around 2.5 minutes (about a half mile for a fast runner). That means, for fast people at least, the half mile run is about half aerobic, half anaerobic. Realize, it's not half way on anaerobic, then the other half on aerobic, it's a continuous combination of pathways.

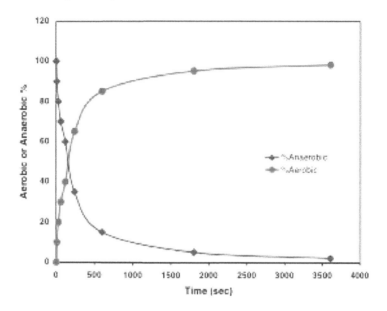

FIGURE 2–4. The percent contributions of aerobic and anaerobic ATP production to maximum sustainable exercise from three seconds to one hour.

Data from Powers and Howley, Exercise Physiology, 5th ed, 2004.

Assignment 2–10. Note that the x-axis for Figure 2.4 is in seconds. Convert the seconds to time frames that you can think about intuitively (for example, minutes). What types of sports/exercise correspond to the different plotted points? For example, think about types of exercise that require only 3–10 sec to complete compared to those that take an hour or more. Provide an example (write down) for at least seven of the nine time points.

Part 3. Skeletal Muscle

Muscle is a popular topic. If you walk through a grocery store or an airport, you can find lots of magazines full of tips on how to get more of it. Of course, these magazines are focused on skeletal muscle, the muscles found in association with bones and joints. There are two other types of muscle—cardiac and smooth, which serve critical autonomic (like, automatic) functions such as blood circulation and digestion. In this class, we will focus on skeletal muscle, but cardiac and smooth muscle are discussed in other classes, such as anatomy and physiology, human physiology, and exercise testing and prescription.

Muscle Macroscopic Anatomy

On average, muscles make up 30% or more of a person's total body mass. Men have a higher absolute and relative body weight as muscle than do women. The gender differences are greater in the upper body than the lower, which corresponds to the greater disparity in upper body strength, compared to lower body strength, between men and women.

Introduction to Exercise Science is not focused on anatomy, but to become conversant in exercise science, athletic training, or human biology, it is necessary to know (off hand) the names of major skeletal muscles in the body. You should know the locations and actions of at least the following muscles: masseter, deltoid, pectoralis major, biceps brachii, triceps brachii, brachioradialis, rectus abdominis, diaphragm, vastus group (lateralis, intermedius, medialis), gluteus maximus, hamstring group (semimembranosus, semitendinosus, biceps femoris), gracilis, gastrocnemius, soleus, and tibialis anterior. You can find all of these muscles (and many more!) on labeled diagrams in textbooks and online.

Backtracking to the Somatic Nervous System

Before we continue on to muscle cell structure and function, we will backtrack a bit and discuss the nervous activation of muscle. The entirety of your nervous system can be divided into central and peripheral. The central nervous system (often abbreviated CNS) consists of your brain and spinal cord. That is easy to remember. Everything else is in the peripheral nervous system. Peripheral nerves can be divided by directionality—those taking information TO the CNS, and those taking information FROM the CNS. The nerves taking information to the spinal cord and brain are sensory nerves, also known as afferent nerves. The nerves taking information from the CNS are motor nerves, also known as efferent (e, like "exit") nerves. Among the motor nerves, there are two types—somatic and autonomic. The somatic motor nerves go to skeletal muscles. As you know, skeletal muscles are voluntary, meaning, you can control them by willful thought. The autonomic motor nerves go to the muscles you can't control by thought—the cardiac and smooth muscles that function "automatically." For the rest of our discussion on nerves, we will focus on only the somatic motor neurons. You will discuss nerves in greater breadth and detail in classes such as anatomy and physiology.

Assignment 2–11.   Diagram the nervous system, showing the CNS, peripheral nervous system, sensory nerves, motor nerves, autonomic motor nerves, and somatic motor nerves.

Neuromuscular Junction

A neuron is a single nerve cell (nerves are comprised of many individual cells). Each neuron has a cell body that contains the usual organelles—nucleus, mitochondria, endoplasmic reticulum, etc. Emanating from the cell body of a somatic motor neuron is a long skinny shaft—the axon. The axon may be quite long (like a long hair), but is far, far thinner than a human hair. The axon branches at the end and each branch extends to a single muscle cell. Note, each motor neuron extends branches to multiple (could be 100+) muscle cells. One motor neuron plus all of the muscle cells associated with its axon is called a motor unit. The place where the motor neuron's branch and the muscle cell *almost* meet is called the neuromuscular junction. The small gap between the end of the axon and the muscle cell membrane is called the neuromuscular cleft or synapse. In our world, it is an infinitesimal space, but in the world of molecules, it's like the Mississippi river.

In order for a neuron to initiate a contraction in a muscle cell, the neuron must send a message through the synapse to the muscle cell. This message takes the form of a substance known as a neurotransmitter (neuro like neuron, transmitter like transmitter). There are many different kinds of neurotransmitters, but the one used by a somatic motor neuron is called acetylcholine, abbreviated ACH. The ACH sails the synapse and docks at the muscle cell. It does not enter the muscle cell, rather, it binds to a receptor that is on the outer surface of the muscle cell. A receptor is analogous to a little catcher's mitt, except receptors are specific. ACH has its own receptor. Other neurotransmitters, as well as hormones like insulin, have their own receptors. The binding of ACH to its receptor sets off a chain reaction, like knocking down the first domino in a series. These changes include a change in the ion permeability of the muscle cell. Specifically, channels for sodium ions (Na^+) open. Sodium enters the cell for two reasons: It enters because doing so involves moving from high to low concentration, and it enters because the inside of the cell is negatively charged, while sodium ions are positively charged. After enough sodium ions enter, the inside of the cell becomes positively charged. This electrical shift inside the cell from negative to positive is termed depolarization. The entire process is also called an action potential.

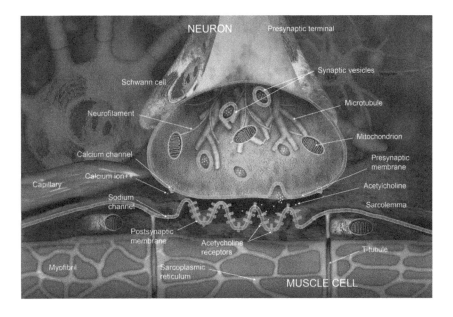

FIGURE 2–5. Neuromuscular junction.

Visuals Unlimited, Inc./Carol and Mike Werner.

The changes in membrane permeability are not limited to opening of sodium channels. Channels for other ions, such as potassium (K^+) are also opened, and the end result is that an action potential comes and goes rapidly. The cell quickly repolarizes, meaning, a negative charge is re-established inside the cell.

After we have discussed the microstructure of a muscle cell, we will return to what is known as excitation—contraction coupling, or in other words, we will cover how the electrical changes lead to force generation ("pull") by the muscle cell.

Muscle Microscopic Anatomy

Muscle cells do not look like the stereotypical "fried egg" cell that is illustrated in basic biology texts. Certainly, muscle cells, also known as "fibers," do have most of the same organelles, such as nuclei, mitochondria, golgi, etc., however, they have them in different proportions than many cells. Furthermore, as you might imagine, skeletal muscle cells are long and thin, not round or column shaped. Like other cells, the muscle cell is enclosed by a membrane. This membrane is called the sarcolemma. The prefix "sarco" indicates muscle. In other cells, the outer membrane is called the plasmalemma. The sarcolemma has multiple, deep, invaginations. To envision these invaginations, think of a bowling ball. A bowling ball is round and smooth on the outside, except where the finger holes are. If you submerge the bowling ball in water, the water will touch the entire surface, including inside the holes. Muscle cells have multiple holes like the finger holes on the bowling ball, and they are called T-tubules. The T-tubules allow the surface (plasma membrane) to extend deep into the muscle, like the finger holes in a bowling ball. In physiology, you will find multiple biological techniques for expanding surface area—the T-tubules are one example.

A muscle cell does not have one nucleus. It has many. Many can mean a dozen or even a hundred! Some of the nuclei are deep inside the cell, but many are right under the sarcolemma (near the cell surface). Having multiple nuclei is a little bit like having many brains. Muscle cells can have sort of "split personalities." We'll return to that thought later. Muscle cells also have mitochondria, organelles we mentioned in the bioenergetics section. Like the nuclei, some of the mitochondria are deep in the cell, and others are subsarcolemmal. Muscle cells have endoplasmic reticulum, only, it's called sarcoplasmic reticulum. The sacroplasmic reticulum and T-tubules form structural triads—one T-tubule with sacroplasmic reticulum on two sides. The sacroplasmic reticulum functions as a storage depot for calcium ions (Ca^{++}). That means that the concentration of calcium ions inside the sacroplasmic reticulum is high—higher than that inside the rest of the cell.

Muscle cells also have the structures necessary for contraction and force generation. In fact, these proteins take up most of the space inside the cell. The two most fundamental contractile proteins are actin and myosin. Actin is known as the thin filament because it is a thin protein, while myosin is known as the thick filament because it is thicker. (This concept is no more difficult than thin rope versus fat rope.) Actin and myosin are organized into repeating units known as sarcomeres. In two dimensions, a sarcomere has two ends, known as Z-lines. The actin filaments are bound to the z-lines. The myosin filaments are between the actin filaments. The myosin protein has structures that are called heads, but function like arms. The myosin heads can bind to actin and pull on it. When a myosin head pulls on actin, the Z-lines are drawn closer together. That, fundamentally, is muscle contraction.

Use the many (many!) images of sarcomeres online to make your own diagram. Make sure you have labeled the Z-lines, actin, and myosin.

In very close physical association with the actin are two other "leading role" proteins, tropomyosin and troponin. The tropomyosin is a ribbon-like protein that runs the length of the actin and blocks the sites where myosin could bind to actin, like a socket cover. The troponin can bind calcium. And this brings us back to excitation—contraction coupling.

Excitation-Contraction Coupling

Remember that a motor neuron is required to activate a skeletal muscle cell (note, the same is NOT true for cardiac or smooth muscle cells). When a somatic motor neuron releases ACH, it will excite all of the muscle cells in that motor unit. Excitation involves ion fluxes that lead to the depolarization (negative to positive electrical shift) of the muscle cell. Positive charge inside the cell causes voltage-gated calcium channels on the sarcoplasmic reticulum (SR) to open. (The voltage is related to the charge, so these channels are closed when the cell is negative inside.) Because the calcium is very concentrated inside the SR, the calcium falls out, like toys falling out of an over-stuffed closet. Some of those calcium ions encounter troponin. When troponin binds the calcium, the three dimensional shape of the protein changes, which in turn causes a change in the tropomyosin protein. The shift in the tropomyosin exposes the myosin binding sites on the actin. The myosin heads may now bind.

Sacromeres exist in both parallel (next to each other) and series (one after another). When lots of myosin heads pull on lots of actin molecules at once, the entire muscle cell is undergoing a contraction. Depending on the nature of the contraction, the cell may or may not get shorter, which may seem like a paradoxical statement. A little further along, we'll discuss how contraction of a muscle cell does not always mean the cell gets shorter.

Muscle contraction would be no fun at all without muscle relaxation. Simple movements like walking and breathing involve alternating contraction and relaxation of multiple muscle groups. Muscle relaxation is more or less the reverse of contraction. The calcium must un-bind from the troponin, causing the myosin binding sites to be again obstructed. To achieve this, pumps on the sarcoplasmic reticulum surface move calcium "uphill," back into the sarcoplasmic reticulum. These pumps require ATP to operate (just like pumps moving water uphill require electricity). So, take note, *energy is required for muscle relaxation.*

As you might guess, energy is also required for contraction. When the myosin heads bind actin, an ATP is used to achieve the "pull" on the actin (the force generation). In addition, an ATP is required to get the myosin off the actin—either for relaxation OR for further contraction. If each myosin bound to actin and pulled only once, the muscle would hardly shorten at all. Instead, the myosin must move on to the next actin binding site, and pull again, and again. This is called cross-bridge cycling. The bond between myosin and actin is the cross-bridge, and the cycling refers to the process of bind-pull-release-bind-pull-release. To get a sense of what this is like, think of pulling on a rope with one hand only. You would reach out, grab the rope, and pull. If you only have one hand available, in order to pull more, you will need to release the rope, grab at a new spot, and pull again.

Assignment 2–13. Make an ordered list of the steps needed for excitation-contraction coupling. Start with the release of ACH from the motor neuron and finish with muscle contraction then relaxation. You should include at least nine steps.

Assignment 2–14. Research an example of a disease or poison that affects excitation-contraction coupling. Any part of the process, from the motor neuron to the sarcomere may be affected. Write down the name of the disease/poison, the symptoms, and explain the physiology—what is affected and how.

Types of Skeletal Muscle

Depending on the work expected of them, skeletal muscle cells differ in their structural and biochemical complement. Some muscle cells are needed for fast, strong contractions. Others are needed for more sustained or repeated contractions over a long period of time. Consider the difference between standing or walking, and a bench press or high jump. Standing requires the postural muscles to sustain contraction for as long as you want to stay standing (which sometimes, such as at the airport, can be a while). Walking on campus from one building to another requires repeated contraction-relaxation cycles of several muscles. A bench press or high jump, however, requires one fast, high force contraction (of several muscles). To accommodate these different activities, there are three* basic types of muscle.

TABLE 2–2. Three basic types of skeletal muscle

Type	Alternate name	Example
Type I	Slow oxidative	Soleus
Type IIa	Fast oxidative-glycolytic OR Intermediate	Vastus lateralis
Type IIb	Fast glycolytic	Tibialis anterior

Keep in mind that entire muscles (e.g., soleus, vastus lateralis, tibialis anterior, biceps brachii, etc.) generally have individual cells of all three types. But some muscles have more of one type than another, for example the soleus is ~90% slow oxidative.

The equipment and capacities of these three fiber types differ. As you might imagine, the slow muscle contracts more slowly than the fast muscle. The slow oxidative muscle uses predominantly oxidative phosphorylation for ATP generation, so it has a lot of mitochondria. Since aerobic ATP generation is more efficient than anaerobic, slow oxidative muscle is more efficient and is less fatigable than the more glycolytic types. The fast glycolytic (Type IIb) muscle has the fewest mitochondria and the least resistance to fatigue, however it is the fastest. Type IIa is intermediate in most respects—it is faster than slow, but not as fast as IIb, it is more aerobic than IIb, but less aerobic than slow oxidative, and so forth. In general, the blood supply to slow oxidative fibers is greater than that to fast glycolytic fibers—can you speculate on why that is so?

TABLE 2-3. Characteristics of Different Muscle Fiber Types

Type	Speed	Metabolism	Mitochondria	Efficiency	Endurance	Size
I	Slow	Oxidative	Most	Best	Greatest	Smallest
IIa	Fast	Mixed	Many	Medium	Medium	Intermediate
IIb	Fastest	Glycolytic	Least	Least	Least	Largest

Muscle Plasticity

One of the neat things about muscle is that it is not non-malleable, but rather it is what physiologists call "plastic." Plastic is flexible, and indeed, the muscle cells are flexible in the sense that they can change. Muscle cells can grow bigger (a characteristic that provides the ultimate source material for quite a few popular magazines). Use will stimulate muscle cells to get bigger, a process known as **hypertrophy**. Hyper means "above," trophy refers to growth. So, it's growth above and beyond regular somatic (child to adult) growth. The capacity of muscle cells to grow is essential, because muscle cells rarely (if ever) divide. So, with very rare exception, adults cannot gain more muscle by hyperplasia (addition of new cells). Muscle cells can also get smaller with lack of use, and that is termed **atrophy**. Atrophy of muscles is a problem for space station astronauts, due to the lack of gravity in space and limited opportunities for exercise. Bed rest, casts (such as after a broken bone is set), and spinal cord injury can also lead to muscle atrophy.

In addition to changing size, muscle cells can also change their biochemical composition, meaning, they can become more or less aerobic with changes in enzyme ratios. They can also become faster or slower with changes in proteins such as myosin. Aerobic exercise training will stimulate Type IIb fibers to transform into more aerobic Type IIa fibers. More aerobic training might even stimulate some Type IIa fibers to become slow oxidative Type I fibers. The opposite changes are also possible. Disuse, as described above, will lead to a transformation of Type IIa fibers into Type IIb fibers. The fact that fibers can change type suggests that there can be in-between or transitional states. Indeed, these are seen—fibers that are somewhere between the discrete types. This fact brings us back to the multiple nuclei. Some nuclei can be directing cellular function according to one type, while others are acting like another type—at the same time. So, back when I first introduced the three types of skeletal muscle, I put a star next to three. That's because in reality, muscle cells do not necessarily all fall within one of these three discrete categories, just like in reality, not everyone has exactly blue or exactly brown eyes—there's bright blue and grayish blue, hazel and green, and black (I think black is only for vampires). But, just because there are shades of blue and shades of brown, we don't ditch the concept of blue eyes versus brown. Likewise, we're not going to toss the three types scheme just because nature is less rigid.

You might think that resistance (like weight) training would lead to a conversion of Type IIa to Type IIb fibers, since resistance training is largely anaerobic. However, resistance training does not cause this transition, in fact, the opposite. The bottom line is that USE (exercise, of any type) tends to cause a more aerobic muscle profile. In the case of endurance training, Type I fibers are emphasized. Resistance training leads to an increase in both size and percentage of Type IIa fibers. Only lack of use (including deprivation of neural input as in spinal cord injury) leads to an increase in the percentage of Type IIb fibers.

Are people all born with the same muscle composition? Of course not. If you look at a mixed muscle such as the vastus lateralis or gastrocnemius, you will see different percentages of the three fiber types in different individuals. So while training can influence muscle size and biochemistry, genetics also plays a role.

TABLE 2–4. Percentages of Type I, IIa, and IIb fibers in the thigh muscle of endurance athletes, power athletes, and untrained individuals.

Sport Status	Type I (Slow ox)	Type IIa (FOG)	Type IIb (Fast gly)
Distance runners	63–71%	29–31%	1–6%
Power lifters	53%	46%	1%
Sedentary (untrained)	55%	33%	12%

Data on distance runners from Harber et al., 02; Kyrolainen et al., 03; Kohn et al. 07.
Data on power lifters and sedentary people from Fry et al., 2004.

Assignment 2–15.   We all know that men are stronger than women. The difference in strength is more pronounced for upper body activities (e.g., bench press) than lower body activities (e.g., leg press). Explain the physiological basis for the strength differences between men and women. Are the differences at the subcellular, cellular, or macroscopic level?

Types of Muscle Contraction

The stereotypical muscle contraction is one in which the muscle produces force as it gets shorter. However, you can try a simple exercise (or two) to demonstrate to yourself that muscles can "contract" (be active) but not shorten. First, try putting your hands together, palm to palm, in front of you and push with each hand on the other. You should feel muscle contraction, but neither hand moves, and hence in neither arm is muscle shortening. Consider also the standard biceps curl exercise. Put a dumbbell weight (a milk container or heavy book will suffice as well) in each hand, with your arms resting at your sides. Now, bend your elbows to "curl" the weight up toward your chest. Your biceps produced force and became shorter as you flexed your elbow; this is a standard (concentric) contraction. But what about lowering the weight? If you lower it slowly, your biceps will do work as it lengthens. If you aren't sure that your biceps is doing work, then I recommend you go to a gym, get a moderately heavy weight, and do this exercise over and over. You can even skip the elbow flexing (weight up) part—have a friend do that. Just lower the weight over and over. See how your biceps feels in a day or two. I suspect then you will know that your muscle did work.

So, the muscle can be active when there is no change in length, when it shortens, or as it lengthens. These three muscle actions are called isometric, concentric, and eccentric contractions, in that order. You may also occasionally see reference to isotonic or isokinetic contractions. Isotonic means that the force of the contraction remains constant, and isokinetic means that the speed of rotation (e.g., rotation around the elbow or knee) remains constant. There are special machines, used particularly in athletic training rehabilitation or physical therapy settings, that force an isokinetic contraction. See if someone you know has used one of these machines. Ask that person how the motion felt.

Properties of Skeletal Muscle Contraction

There are a couple of interesting rules for skeletal muscle contraction. The first is that for a given fiber (muscle cell), there is a speed-force trade off, also called the force-velocity curve. As the speed of contraction gets faster, the maximum force possible gets lower. The opposite is also true—as the contraction becomes slower, the maximum force gets higher. Thus, the force produced during an isometric contraction (no change in length, hence zero speed) is greater than that produced during a faster concentric contraction. Another interesting property is known as the length-tension curve. For any given fiber, there is an optimal length for force production. If the fiber is stretched above the optimal length (note—if your biceps brachii contracts, the triceps is stretched. If the triceps contracts, the biceps is stretched), the force is reduced. If the cell is not stretched enough (too slack, essentially), the force is also reduced. The optimal length is really a range of intermediate levels of stretch. The reason for the length-tension curve can be understood at the molecular level. Within each sarcomere, there is an optimal level of actin and myosin overlap. If the sarcomere is stretched too far, some of the myosin heads cannot reach an actin molecule and the number of cross-bridges formed is thereby reduced. If there is too much overlap, multiple myosin heads compete for the same actin binding sites, and again, fewer cross-bridges are produced. Force ultimately comes down to cross-bridges—more cross-bridges will combine to produce greater force.

Loss of Muscle Mass with Aging

Most people maintain muscle mass until about the forth or fifth decade. At some point, muscle mass, and consequently strength, start to decline. This is true in both men and women, in fact, it may be slightly more pronounced in men. Sarcopenia is the term that was invented to describe "clinically" low levels of muscle. Since muscle strength is correlated with mass, a low muscle mass can lead to inadequate strength for daily living activities such as getting in and out of cars, lifting groceries, etc. You already know that disuse will lead to a loss in muscle mass. Disuse likely contributes to muscle loss with aging as people tend to become less active, particularly in their 70's and 80's. Disuse does not explain all of the loss in muscle mass and strength with aging, however, as even master athletes are affected, despite training as much as their younger counterparts. Both the number of motor units and the number of muscle cells themselves decline in people as they age beyond about 50 years. The reasons for loss in muscle number and mass are not all known, but hormonal changes likely contribute. Growth hormone is essential for normal child to adult growth, and is a player in maintaining both muscle and bone mass in adulthood. Growth hormone pulses decrease in amplitude (pulses get smaller) as we age. Levels of sex steroids (testosterone, estrogen) also tend to decrease as we age. Most people have heard of menopause, after which sex steroid levels in women are markedly reduced. Fewer people realize that many older men have low (compared to younger men) levels of testosterone. These factors and others may contribute to sarcopenia.

The good news is that older people can improve muscle strength with resistance training. In general, men respond more robustly than women—absolute gains are larger. However, anyone can benefit from strength training.

References

Harber M. P, Gallagher P. M, Trautmann J, Trappe S. W. 2002. "Myosin Heavy Chain Composition of Single Muscle Fibers in Male Distance Runners." *Int J Sports Med* 23 (7):484–88.

Jackson, D. C. 1987. "Assigning Priorities Among Interacting Physiological Systems." In: *New Directions in Ecological Physiology.* M. E. Feder, A.F. Bennett, W. W. Burggren, and R. B. Huey, eds., Cambridge, MA: Cambridge Univ. Press, pp. 310–26,

Kyrolainen H, Kivela R, Koskinen S, McBride J, Andersen J. L, Takala T, Sipila S, Komi P. V. 2003. Interrelationships "Between Muscle Structure, Muscle Strength, and Running Economy." *Med Sci Sports Exerc.* 35 (1):45–49.

Powers, S. K. and Howley, E. T. *Exercise Physiology,* 5th ed. 2004. McGraw-Hill.

Chapter 3

CARDIOVASCULAR AND PULMONARY PHYSIOLOGY

Part 1. Cardiovascular Physiology

Intuitively, cardiovascular physiology features quite prominently in exercise physiology. If you take the name apart, you can identify the two components we will address—the heart (cardio) and blood vessels (vasculature). This chapter will cover the fundamental physiology from which all of the complex functions follow. Cardiovascular physiology is discussed in greater depth in courses such as anatomy and physiology, exercise physiology, human or animal physiology, and exercise testing and prescription.

Cardiac Anatomy

Before we can discuss how the heart works, you need a basic concept of cardiac anatomy. Mammals have four chambered hearts, arranged in a two-by-two organization (two chambers on the left, two on the right). Each chamber has an inflow and an outflow. The left side of the heart is known as the "systemic" side. It pumps blood out to the body. The right side of the heart is known as the "pulmonary" side. It pumps blood to the lungs.

Assignment 3–1.   Find an illustration of human cardiac anatomy. Use the illustration to identify the following structures: right atrium, right AV valve, right ventricle, pulmonary artery, pulmonary valve, pulmonary vein, left atrium, left AV (mitral) valve, left ventricle, aorta, aortic valve, superior vena cava, inferior vena cava, sino-atrial (SA) node, atrio-ventricular (AV) node. You will be asked in class and on quizzes or exams to draw the heart and label all these structures from memory.

Vascular Anatomy

The vasculature is ultimately a loop—vertebrates have what is called a "closed" circulatory system. If you follow the path of a single blood cell around the body, you can see that it always returns to the point where it started. The closed nature of the vasculature was not always known—because the smallest blood vessels are microscopic, for a long time, people did not know they existed. For 1400 years, the opinion of Galen (129–207 AD), one of the most famous ancient physicians, prevailed. He said that blood was created in the liver and consumed at the tissues—a one-way street. In 1628, William Harvey published his now famous text on the circulatory system, which is much closer to our current view. He deduced the existence of capillaries, which were discovered in 1660 by Marcello Malpighi with the aid of a microscope (Lubitz, 2004).

Five categories of blood vessel will be described—arteries, arterioles, capillaries, venules, and veins. The largest artery in the body is the aorta, which is roughly 2.5 cm in diameter. Arteries carry blood away from the heart and are essentially high pressure tubing. They have relatively thick, resilient walls. If an artery is smaller than 0.03 mm in diameter, it is called an arteriole. Arterioles are known as "stopcock" vessels. They are wrapped with smooth muscle that can, by contracting and constricting the vessel, decrease the diameter. Conversely, if the smooth muscle is relaxed, the arteriole is open as widely as possible. In this way, arterioles exert control over the distribution of blood flow throughout the body. You need a system that can increase or decrease blood flow to different areas because, for example, when you run, your leg muscles need more blood than they do at rest; when you eat, your digestive tract needs more. (What happens when you eat and then run?)

Arterioles feed into capillaries. Capillaries, as previously mentioned, are so small they can only be seen with a microscope. Capillary diameter is approximately 0.008 mm. The walls of capillaries are also very thin—one cell thick, in fact. The capillaries have no extras—no smooth muscle or extra connective tissue. The minimalistic barrier is essential because capillaries are the site where oxygen and nutrients exit the blood and go into the tissue cells (like muscle cells). Likewise, carbon dioxide and other wastes exit body cells and enter the blood at the capillaries. Although the size of any one capillary is tiny, there are so many capillaries that the total (integrated) cross-sectional area is huge—500 times that of the aorta. Why is such a large surface area needed?

Capillaries lead to venules, which in turn lead to veins. Venules are roughly 0.02 mm in diameter, while the largest veins, the superior and inferior vena cavae, are about 3 cm in diameter. Veins are called "capacitance" vessels. They are distensible (if you don't recognize that word, look it up) and that provides for the capacity. When you are resting (sitting in class, watching TV etc.), about two-thirds of your total blood volume is contained in the veins. If you exercise, that percentage will be reduced. A unique feature of veins is the one-way valves. One way valves are like saloon doors—they can be pushed open in one direction, but not the other. These valves will open only in the direction toward the heart. That way, if you go from lying down to standing, all the blood in your veins doesn't fall into your feet!

Blood is under pressure in the arteries—in fact, that is what we call arterial blood pressure, and it's what you have measured when you go to a doctor's office. The pressure drops throughout the circuit such that the pressure in the large veins is very low—0 to 2 mmHg. If you cut a vein, blood will drip, drip, drip out. If you cut an artery, the blood might very well hit the ceiling! The drop in pressure from artery to vein is not evenly distributed throughout the circuit—most of the drop takes place in the arterioles. Think about it—would you want a high pressure in the very thin walled capillaries? In addition, the flow goes from pulsatile (due to the beating of the heart) to continuous in the arterioles. It is normal to feel a pulse in larger arteries such as the carotid in your neck or the radial artery in your wrist. It is not normal to feel a pulse in veins.

Assignment 3–2.   Arteries take blood away from the heart. Veins return blood to the heart. There are no exceptions. Arteries carry oxygenated, red, arterial blood. There is one exception. Veins carry deoxygenated, bluer, venous blood. There is one exception. Given what you have studied so far, identify the two aforementioned exceptions.

Cardiac Output

Fundamentally, the heart is a pump. It's job is to move blood at a sufficient rate and in sufficient quantity to keep the body tissues supplied with oxygen and nutrients. Exercise increases the rate at which the body uses oxygen and nutrients, and therefore increases the load on the heart. We measure the output of the heart in liters of blood pumped out per minute. This measure is called the cardiac output. Maximum cardiac output is the maximum pump capacity of the heart—the best it can do. Maximum cardiac output is an extremely important clinical measure and also an important measure in endurance athletes. Cardiac output is the multiplicative product of two factors—the heart rate (beats per minute) and the stroke volume, which is the volume (liters or ml) of blood ejected with each beat.

$$Q \text{ (L/min)} = HR \text{ (beats/min)} * SV \text{ (L/beat)}$$

You must commit this simple equation to memory. This equation should also make sense to you. Think about the following analogy. If you were in the shipping business, you might have a set number of trucks available to you. Let's say you had 10 trucks. Each truck can be loaded with up to 12 tons of your goods (oranges or paper clips or solar panels). If demand is low, you might send out only five trucks per day, each loaded at half capacity. That's five trucks/day times six tons/truck, for a total of 30 tons sent out per day. Let's say demand increases. Now you might add a sixth truck and send them all out fully loaded. Now you have six trucks/day times 12 tons/truck, for a total of 72 tons sent out per day. You can move up to maximum capacity (all 10 trucks, all fully loaded). Cardiac output is the same idea. You can increase the frequency (number of beats in a minute—analogous to trucks per day) and you can increase the volume in each beat (liters in each beat-analogous to the tons on each truck) up to a maximum.

Assignment 3–3.   The ability to raise cardiac output is an important clinical index (relates to a patient's prognosis). If a patient has a resting heart rate of 70 bpm and has the capacity to reach 130 bpm, and a resting stroke volume of 50 ml/beat and can raise it to 90 ml/beat, by how many L/min can he raise his cardiac output?

Control of Heart Rate

Unlike skeletal muscle, cardiac muscle will contract even in the absence of neural input. This fact has been grotesquely illustrated in movies such as Indiana Jones and the Temple of Doom, when one of the nasty characters rips the heart out of a live person, and the disembodied heart continues to beat in the bad guy's hand. The inherent pace of the heart is set by a group of "pacemaker" cells in the SA node. You should have found the SA node in your anatomy research. The pacemaker cells are leaky to sodium. Sodium leaks in and eventually causes an action potential. That excitation is then propagated to other heart muscle cells and the muscle of the atria contract in unison, and then, after a very short lag, the muscle of the ventricles contract in unison.

Autonomic (not somatic) motor nerves extend to the SA node and can increase or decrease the heart rate by affecting the pacemaker cells. The cardiac accelerator nerve is part of the sympathetic nervous system. As the name indicates, it can act to increase heart rate. It does this by releasing nor-epinephrine, a hormone/neurotransmitter you may know better by the name of "nor-adrenaline." The counter to the sympathetic nervous system is called the parasympathetic nervous system. Within that system, a nerve called the Vagus nerve extends to the heart and can slow heart rate by releasing ACH. The sympathetic and parasympathetic nervous systems work together, like yin and yang, to control heart rate and many other bodily functions. The sympathetic nervous system is dominant in "flight or fight" situations—situations when you'd expect to have a racing heart! In contrast, the parasympathetic nervous system is dominant in "eat or sleep" scenarios, when heart rate is slow. Under typical conditions, the parasympathetic nervous system is braking heart rate—the inherent rate of the pacemaker cells is higher than what you observe. During high intensity exercise, heart rate may be at its maximum. Maximum heart rate is not clearly related to fitness or gender, but it is related to age. Older people have lower maximum heart rates. For adults, a useful heuristic is 220 minus age. So, for example, the estimated maximum heart rate of a 20 year-old is 200 beats per minute.

Control of Stroke Volume

The control of stroke volume is more complex than that of heart rate. There are three basic factors that affect stroke volume: preload, afterload, and contractility. Preload is the amount of blood in the ventricles just prior to contraction. The basic mantra here is 'if you put more in, you get more out'. This principle is called the Frank-Starling Law, named after two physiologists who described the phenomenon. Venous return of blood fills the ventricles during diastole— the period between heart contractions. For that reason, preload is also called end-diastolic volume (the volume in the ventricles at the end of diastole—just before contraction). If you contract your muscles, by walking around, the muscles press on the veins and squish blood toward the heart (not away, due to the one-way valves). (For a graphic, try filling a straw with milkshake, then put one finger on the bottom of the straw, and with your other hand squeeze the middle of the straw. You should get milkshake coming out of the open end.) Gravity also helps return blood to the heart. The more blood is returned, the greater the preload. The more the ventricles are filled, the greater the stretch on the cardiac muscle cells. These cells respond to the stretch by contracting more forcefully, which leads to a greater ejection, and greater stroke volume. Of course, there is a limit—in pathological states, it is possible for the preload to be too great for the heart to handle. But in general, the greater the preload, the greater the stroke volume.

Afterload is not really an opposite of preload, but it does have the opposite effect—the greater the afterload, the lesser the stroke volume. Afterload is essentially the pressure against which the heart has to push in order to eject blood. In particular, the heart has to open the aortic valve to get blood out through the aorta. So, afterload is the pressure on the other side of the aortic valve—that pressure is related to the arterial blood pressure. Afterload is one reason that high blood pressure increases cardiac work.

Contractility is the force of contraction for any given level of preload, or ventricular stretch. Contractility can be influenced by sympathetic nervous stimulation. With epinephrine, the heart cells will contract more forcefully, thus increasing stroke volume. So, to be clear, increased contractility leads to increased stroke volume.

Assignment 3–4.   Beta blockers are one of the drug types commonly used to treat patients with heart problems. Beta blockers decrease the effect of epinephrine on the heart. How do you expect beta blockers to affect heart rate, stroke volume, and cardiac output during exercise?

Assignment 3–5.   Digitalis and nitroglycerin are two of the oldest (but still used) treatments for heart disease. Do research to find out more about both drugs, including how digitalis and nitroglycerin exert their effects. Relate what you learn to the physiology we have covered. Here are some hints: Digitalis is derived from an ornamental plant called foxglove. Over 200 years ago, it was used to treat what was called "dropsy." Nitroglycerin was used for over 100 years without a clear understanding of how it works. The Nobel Prize in physiology or medicine for 1998 was awarded to the people who uncovered its mechanism. Come to class prepared to discuss your findings.

Blood Pressure

As with any system of fluid in a closed tubing arrangement, there is a measurable pressure within the vessels. Since the fluid in the vasculature is blood, we call this blood pressure. Most often, the term blood pressure is intended to mean the systemic arterial blood pressure. You should recognize that there is also a pulmonary arterial blood pressure—the left (systemic) and right (pulmonary) blood pressures are NOT the same! Blood pressure is typically reported as two values—the **systolic** blood pressure "over" the **diastolic** blood pressure. The systolic pressure is the higher of the two numbers. It represents the pressure in the arteries during systole, or contraction of the ventricles. The diastolic pressure is the pressure in the arteries during diastole, when the ventricles are relaxed and filling. High blood pressure, or **hypertension** (hyper—above; tension—pressure), is a common health problem. Systemic hypertension is defined as a systolic pressure above 140 mmHg and/or a diastolic pressure above 90 mmHg. A normal adult systemic blood pressure is 120/80 or lower. The values between "normal" and "hypertension" are sometimes termed "pre-hypertension." Pulmonary arterial blood pressure is about 75% lower than systemic arterial pressure. Pulmonary hypertension is less common than systemic hypertension, but not less serious. One of the reasons the infamous diet drug "fen-phen" was dangerous and banned was because it increased the consumer's risk of pulmonary hypertension.

Assignment 3–6.
Why does blood pressure matter, anyway? What happens if blood pressure becomes too low? Write down the consequences of **hypo**tension.

Control of Blood Pressure

Intuitively, you know that pressure means the degree to which something is pressing down on something else. For fluid in a tube, the pressure is the degree to which the tube presses down on the fluid, or really, the degree to which the fluid presses on the walls of the tube. To understand the control of blood pressure, first, let's think about a static system (no flow). Let's say you have a balloon filled with water. The more water you put in the balloon, the higher the pressure. If you take a half-filled balloon and transfer all the water in it to a smaller balloon, again, the pressure will be higher. Now, let's move on to a dynamic system (with flow). If you want more water pressure in the shower, one option is to turn up the water flow. (Low flow shower heads sometimes disappoint for this reason—it is impossible to get the flow high enough for satisfying pressure.) The same is true with a hose—a higher flow rate through the hose increases the pressure. A smaller hose diameter will also lead to a higher pressure, as will putting your finger over the hose end and thereby occluding some of the opening. From these everyday-life observations, you have a basic understanding of how blood pressure is controlled. Blood pressure is the product of the cardiac output (that's—flow—Liters/minute) and resistance to flow. The single greatest determinant of resistance to flow is the blood vessel (tube) diameter. Remember, we could change pressure by using a narrower or wider tube. We could also increase pressure by occluding outflow—a way to increase resistance.

Mean Arterial Pressure = Q *TPR

Q = cardiac output and TPR = total peripheral resistance. TPR is the combined resistance in all the blood vessels of the body. It's the integrated resistance to the cardiac output flow. This equation (above) is another you need to commit to memory AND make sure you understand.

As previously mentioned, resistance to flow is largely determined by the diameter of the tube. Most blood vessels can be either constricted (smaller diameter) or dilated (larger diameter). The nicotine in cigarettes potentiates vasoconstriction and increases the risk of hypertension. Other factors also contribute to resistance, including the viscosity of the fluid. As fluid viscosity increases, resistance increases, which will increase pressure. Water and molasses (or corn syrup or pure maple syrup) provide a contrast in viscosity. Molasses has a higher viscosity than water, and it's much harder to move molasses through a straw than water! Blood viscosity can be changed. If you dehydrate, your blood becomes more concentrated and more viscous. People living in "mile high" Denver have (on average) a higher blood viscosity than people living in New Orleans because the higher red blood cell concentration of high altitude residents increases blood viscosity.

Exercise causes changes in both cardiac output and total peripheral resistance. Cardiac output goes up during exercise—the higher the intensity of exercise, the higher the cardiac output (until the maximum is reached). Increased flow increases pressure. However, during exercise, arterioles going to the working muscles dilate, lowering resistance.

Assignment 3–7. Find out what happens to blood pressure during exercise. Does it increase, decrease, or stay the same in healthy humans?

Assignment 3–8. There are numerous pharmaceuticals available to lower blood pressure. Research one—find out the name of the drug (both the "real" name and the marketed name) and basically how it works. Relate the mechanism of action to what you have learned about control of blood pressure. Record and bring to class.

Part 2. Pulmonary Physiology

The incontrovertible association between exercise and increased respiratory effort has been noted since ancient times. Almost 2000 years ago, Galen said " . . . those movements which do not alter the respiration are not called exercise" (from Tipton, 2003). People exercising in a hypoxic (low oxygen) environment may experience a sense of breathlessness, or inability to "catch their breath." The epitome of hypoxic environments is the peak of Mount Everest. Reinhold Messner, who, along with Peter Habler, was the first to summit Everest without supplemental oxygen, said of himself at the summit "I am nothing more than a single narrow gasping lung, floating over the mists and summits."

Functions of Respiration

The most obvious function of respiration is gas exchange. There are two gases of primary concern: oxygen and carbon dioxide. Ventilation makes oxygen available to the body and provides a mechanism for carbon dioxide removal. Respiration has other functions. Tied to the control of carbon dioxide tension (pressure) is acid-base regulation. The link between carbon dioxide and pH is critical to acid-base physiology.

$$CO_2 + H_2O \leftrightarrow H_2CO_3 \leftrightarrow HCO_3^- + H^+$$

Often the unstable intermediate is omitted, leaving:

$$CO_2 + H_2O \leftrightarrow HCO_3^- + H^+$$

This equation indicates that carbon dioxide can combine with water (which is always available in the living body) to form a bicarbonate ion (HCO_3^-) and a proton (H^+). This reaction requires an enzyme, carbonic anhydrase, and takes place inside red blood cells. The relationship of this reaction to blood pH is evident since pH is a measure of the H^+ concentration, converted to a negative log. If removal of carbon dioxide from the body is insufficient, as can be the case in narcotic overdose, then this reaction will go forward and $[H^+]$ will increase, which is known as an acidosis. If more carbon dioxide is removed from the body than is generated by aerobic metabolism, then the reaction will occur in reverse and the [H^+] will decrease, which is known as an alkalosis.

Assignment 3–9.　　You can voluntarily increase or decrease the amount of carbon dioxide in your blood. How do you do that? Write a one sentence plan for each. Describe how blood pH changes in each case.

In addition to gas exchange and contributing to acid-base regulation, respiration also has a role in thermoregulation. This role is particularly important in panting species. Dogs are emblematic panters, but actually atypical. Dogs pant with their mouths open, whereas most animals that pant do so with a closed mouth, passing air over the nasal passages. Panting increases respiratory evaporative water loss, which increases respiratory evaporative heat loss. The role of respiration in human thermoregulation is less obvious, but certainly not non-existent. Ventilatory volume (liters of air per minute) is increased in severely heat-stressed humans, and inversely, ventilatory volume is decreased in hypothermic humans.

Ventilation also indirectly contributes to venous return of blood to the heart. This function will make more sense after we have discussed the mechanics of breathing.

Alternatives to Pulmonary Ventilation

Not all animals have lungs. You already knew that, as I'm sure you figured that worms and sea urchins and bees (for examples) don't have lungs. If you think further, you'll realize that not all vertebrate animals have lungs, since fish and some amphibians have gills. Interestingly, there are amphibians that have neither lungs nor gills. These lungless salamanders achieve gas exchange across their skin. These rather cute amphibians can be found on several continents and quite competently run away when threatened.

Reptiles, birds, and mammals all have lungs. The lungs are less complex in some reptiles, and in the case of snakes, usually there is only one long lung (rather than two). Mammals display what is known as tidal ventilation. Air goes in and out, like tides. Birds do not exhibit tidal ventilation, which provides them some advantages in terms of oxygenating the blood. There are birds that fly over Mount Everest—think about that in the context of Messner's quote at the start of this section.

Anatomy of the Respiratory System

As we did with cardiovascular physiology, we will preface our discussion of physiology with an overview of the anatomy. Fundamentally, there are two parts to the respiratory system, the conducting zone and the respiratory zone. No gas exchange occurs in the conducting zone. The conducting zone is a pipe-way that starts at the nose and mouth and ends at the respiratory ducts. Air travels through the nasal and/or oral cavities to the pharynx, the area where the oral and nasal cavities merge. After passing through the larynx, air enters the trachea. The trachea is a single tube, supported with cartilage C-shaped rings. You can feel these rings in your neck. The open part of the "C" is to the back, or dorsal, side. Near the lungs, the trachea branches into left and right primary bronchi. After that point, the airway branches again and again (on both sides). After 17 branch points (Aykac, 2003), the airways become respiratory ducts that lead to the alveoli. The respiratory ducts plus alveoli are the respiratory zone, where gas exchange occurs.

The left and right lungs are not symmetric. The right lung has three lobes or sections, whereas the left has only two. In some mammals (dogs, e.g.), there is an additional "accessory" lobe of the right lung, which extends over the diaphragm, under the heart. Accessory lobes have also been occasionally described in humans, near the apex of the right lung (not near the diaphragm).

The lungs are surrounded by two layers of membrane known as the pleura. The "potential" space between the pleural membranes is called the pleural space. You may read or hear about "pleural pressure" in physiology classes. Pleural pressure is the pressure between these two membranes, and it can be negative or positive. The lung expands or recoils in response to changes in pleural pressure, which are driven primarily by a muscle called the diaphragm. The diaphragm is a skeletal muscle that separates the thoracic cavity (chest) from the abdominal cavity (belly). It is dome shaped such that the apex or peak is cranial (closer to the head) than the attachments to the ribs. When the diaphragm contracts, it pushes down on the abdomen by flattening the dome.

Assignment 3–10. Find in a book or on line a diagram of respiratory system anatomy. Identify the following features: trachea, larynx, right and left primary bronchi, alveoli, right lung, left lung, pleural membranes, diaphragm.

Gas Exchange in the Lung

Gas exchange (acquisition of oxygen and release of carbon dioxide) occurs in the alveoli of the lung. The alveoli are the spherical endings of the respiratory tree—the ends of the multi-branching pathway. Each person has a tremendous number of alveoli, in the ballpark of 480 million (Ochs et al., 2004). A mere cubic millimeter of lung is estimated to contain 170 alveoli (Ochs et al., 2004). The total surface area dedicated to gas exchange is around 50 to 100 square meters—that's about the area of half a tennis court. Imagine taking a piece of paper the size of a tennis court and scrunching it up and putting it inside a person's chest. That mental exercise should give you some idea of how thin the surface is.

Pulmonary capillaries are juxtaposed to the alveoli. The "blood gas barrier" consists of the alveolar wall, the capillary wall, and a tiny bit of supporting material between those two. The blood gas barrier separates the alveolar air from the blood in the pulmonary capillaries. Therefore, oxygen and carbon dioxide must diffuse across the blood gas barrier, in opposite directions. To facilitate this diffusion, the blood gas barrier must be very thin. In addition, the blood gas barrier must not break—its rupture will lead to blood in the airspace, which is not good! Thoroughbred horses frequently experience pulmonary hemorrhage (bleeding) due to high intensity running. In extreme cases, blood drips out the nose of a horse after a race. In less extreme cases, the presence of red blood cells in the lung air space testifies that bleeding has occurred. As you might imagine, horses do not run well when bleeding into their lungs.

Mechanics of Breathing

In order to understand the mechanics of breathing, it's important to keep in mind a fundamental truth—air flows from areas of high pressure to areas of low pressure. High to low pressure air flow is how we get wind, and it's also how we breathe in and out.

Inspiration is active. Active means that energy is required. To breathe in, the diaphragm, as well as some accessory muscles of breathing, such as the intercostals (inter = between, costal = rib), contract. When the diaphragm contracts, it becomes less dome-shaped and pushes down on the liver and abdominal contents. The other muscles push the ribs and sternum up and out. The effect is something like pulling back a piston in a cylinder. The volume inside the chest increases. According to the ideal gas law (PV = nRT), in a closed system, pressure and volume behave as reciprocals. In other words, since volume in the chest increases, the pressure must decrease. The low pressure inside the lungs relative to outside provides the impetus for air flow into the lungs. Air flows from high to low pressure.

Expiration can be achieved by passive recoil of the lungs. When the diaphragm relaxes, the lungs recoil to their original volume. As lung volume decreases, pressure increases. Air flows out. Expiration can be assisted and sped up by muscular energy investment. You can "push" air out with the intercostal muscles. The "push" creates an even higher pressure in the chest, creating a wider gradient (high versus low pressure) for air flow out of the lungs.

Minute Ventilation

The lung's work, ventilation, is quantified in liters (of air) moved in and out of the lungs per minute. Minute ventilation is the product of respiratory rate (breaths per minute) and tidal volume, which is the liters of air per breath. This formula should look familiar.

$$V_E \text{ (liters/min)} = f \text{ (breaths/min)} * V_T \text{ (liters/breath)}$$

$$V_E = \text{minute ventilation; } f = \text{respiratory rate; } V_T = \text{tidal volume}$$

Here we have a two-for-one deal. The equation for minute ventilation is essentially the same as the formula for cardiac output. Both describe a rate of fluid (blood or air) movement (liters/minute) as the product of a frequency (heart rate or breathing rate) and a volume (stroke volume or tidal volume).

Minute ventilation can be increased by an increase in respiratory rate or tidal volume or both. During exercise, both rate and tidal volume increase.

Respiratory Capacities and Volumes

Pulmonary function testing involves more measures than rate, tidal volume, and minute ventilation. Even if you breathe out as fully as you can, some air remains in the lungs. This unexhalable volume of air is called the residual volume. The residual volume assures that the lungs do not collapse completely no matter how hard you exhale. The residual volume can be lost if the chest wall is pierced, such as by a gunshot or stab wound. A collapsed lung is called a pneumothorax. When President Reagan was shot in a (failed) assassination attempt, he suffered a unilateral (one-sided) pneumothorax. Residual volume is not easy (but not impossible) to measure. The vital capacity, the volume of air that can be voluntarily exhaled after a maximal inhalation, is an easier measure. The residual volume plus the vital capacity equals the total lung capacity—the maximum amount of air that can be contained within the lungs.

Total Lung Capacity = Residual Volume + Vital Capacity

Naturally, larger people have larger lungs and greater total lung capacity than smaller people. In addition, men have slightly larger lungs than woman of a comparable body size.

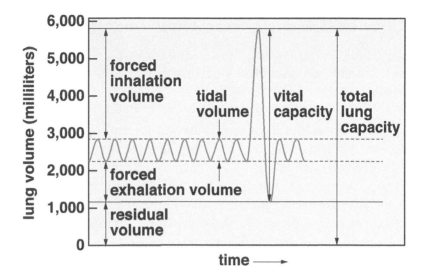

FIGURE 3-1. A spirogram showing tidal volume, residual volume, vital capacity, and total lung capacity.

A measure of particular use in the diagnosis of lung diseases is the forced expiratory volume in one second or FEV1. This measurement is made by asking the subject or patient to breathe in maximally, then breathe out as hard, fast, and fully as possible. Normally, a person can breathe out about 90% of the total exhalation volume (equal to the vital capacity) in the first second of exhalation. If the lungs are compromised such as by chronic obstructive pulmonary disease (COPD), exhalation can become slower and less complete.

Inspired and Alveolar Oxygen Tensions

The primary purpose of breathing is gas exchange. Acquisition of oxygen is one half of this exchange. Oxygen is a component of air. Specifically, oxygen is 20.94% (21%) of air. (The vast majority of the balance is nitrogen.) Air exerts a pressure on the structures around it. At sea level, the air pressure is 1 atmosphere, or 760 mmHg. Per Dalton's law, oxygen provides 21% of that pressure, or 160 mmHg (at sea level).

When a person breathes, air flows through the conducting airways and to the alveoli. As the air travels through the conducting airways, it is humidified, meaning, water vapor is added to the air. The water vapor "bumps" some of the oxygen. The inspired oxygen tension (pressure) is the pressure of oxygen in the humidified air.

$$PIO_2 = (P_B - 47) * 0.21$$

PIO_2 = inspired oxygen tension; P_B = barometric (air) pressure; 47 = vapor pressure of 100% saturated air at 37°F; 0.21 = fraction of oxygen in air.

It is important to note that the inspired oxygen tension is a function of the barometric pressure. Barometric pressure is reduced at high altitude; for example, in Flagstaff, Arizona, the barometric pressure averages around 600 mmHg, in comparison to 760 mmHg at sea level. The saturation vapor pressure at body temperature (37°F) is a constant (doesn't change), and is not a value you need to memorize. The percentage of oxygen in air cannot vary naturally, but can be artificially reduced or increased, and hypoxic or hyperoxic air can be put into tanks.

Assignment 3–11.   Use the equation and values above to calculate the inspired oxygen tension for sea level and for Flagstaff.

When the inspired air flows into the alveoli, a second "bump" occurs. The alveoli are much richer in carbon dioxide than is natural air. The carbon dioxide again displaces some of the oxygen, such that the alveolar oxygen pressure is lower than the inspired oxygen pressure. How much lower depends on the pressure of carbon dioxide in the alveoli. The higher the carbon dioxide pressure, the lower the alveolar oxygen pressure, all other things being equal. The alveolar oxygen pressure sets the upper limit for arterial oxygen pressure. Typically, the arterial oxygen pressure is 3–10 mmHg lower than the alveolar oxygen pressure.

Assignment 3–12.   Explain why the arterial oxygen pressure can never exceed the alveolar oxygen pressure.

Hemoglobin and Oxygen Carrying Capacity

Oxygen diffuses from the air in the alveoli and into the blood; however, oxygen is not very soluble in warm water. That property means that the amount of oxygen that will dissolve in blood is insufficient to sustain endotherms like mammals. Accordingly, most vertebrates and all endotherms have a special carrier for oxygen: the protein hemoglobin. Hemoglobin is contained within the red blood cells. Oxygen diffuses into red blood cells and becomes bound by hemoglobin.

Each hemoglobin molecule contains four binding sites for oxygen. Each binding site contains an iron atom, hence the relationship between iron and oxygen carrying capacity. The *saturation* of hemoglobin with oxygen is quantified as a percentage. If all four binding sites on hemoglobin are bound to oxygen, the hemoglobin is 100% saturated. If three of four sites are bound to oxygen, the hemoglobin is 75% saturated, etc. The arterial blood oxygen saturation (SaO_2) is the average saturation of all the hemoglobin molecules, and theoretically can range from 0% to 100%. At sea level, in healthy, resting adults, the SaO_2 is generally 97% to 99%. Hemoglobin saturation is a function of the blood oxygen tension, but the relationship is not linear.

Assignment 3–13.   Find in a book or on line a graph of the oxy-hemoglobin dissociation curve, i.e., a graph of the relationship between blood oxygen tension and hemoglobin saturation. What shape is the curve? What happens to hemoglobin saturation if oxygen tension drops from 99 mmHg to 90 mmHg? What if it drops from 99 mmHg to 50 mmHg? How does oxygen tension vary between arteries and veins? How does saturation vary between arteries and veins?

Assignment 3–14.   What is myoglobin? Where is it found? What does it do?

Carbon Dioxide Transport in Blood

The other half of gas exchange is the elimination of carbon dioxide. Carbon dioxide is produced by cells engaging in aerobic metabolism. Carbon dioxide diffuses out of these cells and into blood. About 10% of the carbon dioxide is simply dissolved in the blood (the way carbon dioxide is dissolved in a "carbonated" soda). Another roughly 20% of the carbon dioxide binds to hemoglobin inside red blood cells. Finally, the majority of the carbon dioxide, about 70%, is converted inside red blood cells into bicarbonate and H^+ via the reaction delineated at the start of this section. In these three forms, carbon dioxide is transported to the lung. At the lung, dissolved carbon dioxide comes out of solution and diffuses into the alveolar air space. Likewise, carbon dioxide bound to hemoglobin unbinds and diffuses into the alveoli. Finally, the conditions at the lung favor the recombination of bicarbonate and H^+ back into carbon dioxide (which diffuses out) and water.

Ventilation and Exercise Intensity

As you know from practical experience, the harder you exercise, the harder you breathe. The relationship is linear, to a point. After that point, commonly called the *ventilatory threshold*, minute ventilation increases out of proportion with exercise intensity. In other words, at intensities above the ventilatory threshold, a person hyperventilates, expelling more carbon dioxide than is produced. In the graph below, exercise intensity is quantified as the oxygen consumption (VO_2). The ventilatory threshold usually occurs at an intensity that elicits 50–70% of a person's maximum oxygen consumption rate.

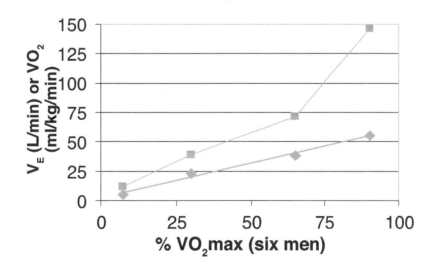

VO$_2$ and V$_E$ by work rate

FIGURE 3–2. Minute ventilation (orange, squares) and oxygen consumption (green, diamonds) plotted as a function of exercise intensity (% maximal oxygen consumption). The ventilatory threshold is seen at an intensity of about 65% of maximum oxygen consumption.

Data from Hopkins et al., 1998.

Assignment 3–15. Use Figure 3–2. Which of the two measurements, minute ventilation or oxygen consumption, is linear over the full range of intensities? Which measurement shows a change in slope? The men hyperventilated at the highest exercise intensity. What change (increase or decrease) in the men's blood pH do you predict occurred at the highest intensity? Justify your answer.

In addition to improving maximal oxygen consumption, aerobic exercise training results in a decrease in the minute ventilation required at a particular oxygen consumption level. Put another way, after training for eight weeks, a person will breathe less hard (lower minute ventilation) than he or she did before training, when running the same speed or producing the same power (watts) on an exercise bicycle. Breathing is essentially more efficient in fitness than in couch-potato-hood.

Assignment 3–16. The male subjects whose data are shown in Figure 3–2 were physically fit. Draw another minute ventilation line for unfit subjects.

References

Hopkins S. R., Gavin T. P., Siafakas N. M., Haseler L. J., Olfert I. M., Wagner H., Wagner P. D. 1998. "Effect of Prolonged, Heavy Exercise on Pulmonary Gas Exchange in Athletes." *J Appl Physiol.* 85 (4):1523–32.

Lubitz S. A., 2004. "Early Reactions to Harvey's Circulation Theory: The Impact on Medicine." *Mt Sinai J Med.* 71:274–80.

Ochs M., Nyengaard J. R., Jung A., Knudsen L., Voigt M., Wahlers T., Richter J., Gundersen H. J. 2004. "The Number of Alveoli in the Human Lung." *Am J Respir Crit Care Med.* 169 (1):120–24.

West J. B. 2003. "Thoughts on the Pulmonary Blood-gas Barrier." *Am. J. Physiol.* 285 (3):L501–13.

Chapter 4

FUNCTIONAL ANATOMY, KINESIOLOGY, AND BIOMECHANICS

Overview and Introduction

The terms Functional Anatomy, Kinesiology, and Biomechanics have been used in many, sometimes interchangeable, ways. Anatomy is the study of the microscopic and macroscopic structure of the body, including muscles, bones, organs and nerves. Functional anatomy, as well as kinesiology, focuses on the use of anatomical features such as bones, tendons and ligaments, to create movement. The terms functional anatomy and kinesiology are often used interchangeably. Kinesiology is also used increasingly in place of the term physical education, and is often used as a substitute for Exercise Science. Therefore, the term kinesiology can be confusing to some. We will use functional anatomy to refer to the function of muscles and their associated bones, tendons, and ligaments in movement. Biomechanics, on the other hand, is less confusing from a terminology sense. In biomechanics, we study the movement itself, the bodies, masses, and forces involved in a resting or moving object.

In this chapter, we will provide an overview of both functional anatomy and biomechanics. This area of study is particularly important to students who plan to become Athletic Trainers, Physical and Occupational Therapists, Physicians and Physician Assistants, as well as anyone who needs to know about the science of movement, including coaches and personal trainers. As you learn about the muscles, joints, and movements discussed in this chapter, apply your understanding of these principles to yourself. Perform the movements mentioned and see how the various muscles act when the joints are moved. Doing this will help you in this class as well as future courses in functional anatomy and biomechanics, as you build a greater level of understanding of movement.

Functional Anatomy

The study of functional anatomy is key to being able to understand and evaluate movement of the body. Movements are initiated and coordinated by the nervous system. The primary work of movement is done by muscles, which respond to signals from the nervous system and pull on the tendons that attach the muscles to the bones. This was discussed in some length in Chapter 3. Also critical in the movement are the bones, on which the muscles act, and the ligaments that attach bone to bone and keep intact the joints that the muscles and tendons cross to allow movement of the body.

Anatomical Position

A standard anatomical position is used as a reference point for describing directions and motions within the body. In the anatomical position, a person stands erect facing forward with feet close together, arms at the side and palms facing forward (Figure 4–1).

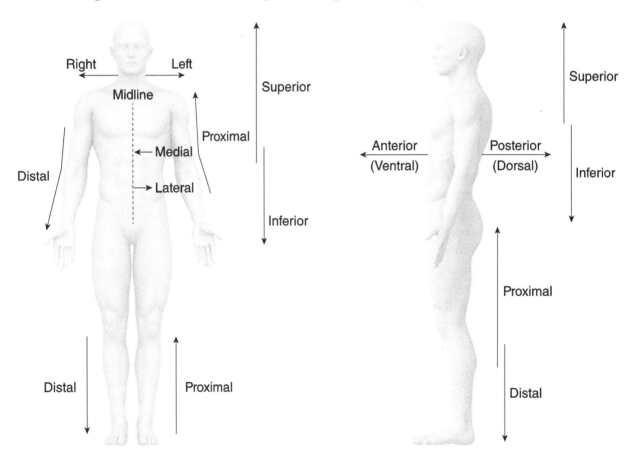

FIGURE 4–1. Person in anatomical position. Directions are also shown in this figure.

In this position, there are many directions, lines, and planes which are used to describe positions and movements. There are six primary directional descriptors:

Anterior: toward the front, also referred to as ventral.

Posterior: toward the back or rear, also termed dorsal.

Superior: toward the head, also referred to as cranial.

Inferior: toward the feet, also called caudal.

Medial: toward the midline of the body.

Lateral: toward the side of the body.

These terms can be combined; for example, the term anterosuperior, means toward the front and head, while posterolateral refers to the outside rear surface.

There are also planes of motion. A plane of motion is an imaginary surface through which a part of the body is moved. There are three cardinal planes, each of which divide the body into two halves (Figure 4–2):

Sagittal: divides the body into right and left halves. Therefore this plane is an anteroposterior plane, meaning it goes from front to back. Movements within this plane are flexion, extension, and hyperextension. An example is the spine. Bending forward is flexion, straightening up is extension, and bending backwards is hyperextension.

Frontal: divides the body into front (anterior or ventral) and back (posterior or dorsal) halves. It is sometimes referred to as the coronal or lateral plane. Movements in the frontal plane are called abduction (moving away from the body) and adduction (moving toward the body). With your arms, bringing them in to your side is adduction, while moving them out from your side is abduction.

Transverse: divides the body into upper (superior or cranial) and lower (inferior or caudal) halves. It is also known as a horizontal or axial plane. Movement within the transverse plane is termed rotation. Simply turning your head is a good example of rotation.

There are also planes termed diagonal or oblique. These are a combination of more than one of the cardinal planes and can be in any number of orientations. In this text, however, we will focus only on the cardinal planes.

Activity 4–1.   Place yourself in anatomical position. Then try movements in the sagittal, frontal and transverse planes. What are examples of these movements that you might perform during a normal day?

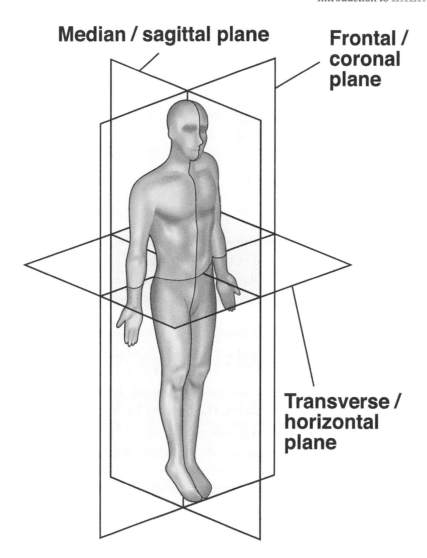

FIGURE 4–2. This shows the three cardinal planes, sagittal, frontal and transverse.
© Kendall Hunt Publishing

The Skeletal System

There are 206 bones that compose the human skeletal system. These bones provide structure to the body to maintain posture, protect the internal organs, serve as attachment points to allow the muscles to produce movement, store minerals (primarily calcium and phosphorus) and produce blood cells. The skeletal system is divided into two portions, the axial skeleton, which consists of the skull, vertebrae, thorax and pelvis, and the appendicular skeleton, or the limbs. For a diagram of the skeleton see Figure 4–3.

Human Skeletal System

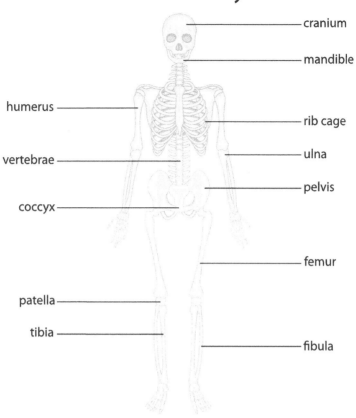

FIGURE 4–3. Diagram of the human skeleton.

© Matthew Cole, 2013. Used under license from Shutterstock, Inc.

Bones can be categorized into one of four major groups based on their shape, long, short, flat, and irregular. **Long bones** include the major bones of the arms and legs, such as the humerus and femur. They have a long shaft with articular surfaces at or near the ends. **Short bones** include the bones of the wrists and ankles, such as the carpal and tarsal bones. **Flat bones** are exemplified by the scapula and sternum. **Irregular bones** are, as named, irregular in shape. The vertebrae are classic examples of irregular bones. In addition, there are bones referred to as **sesamoid bones**. These are bones embedded in tendons. Some authors separate them into a different category, while others do not. The patella is the primary example of a sesamoid bone. See Figure 4–4 for examples of the different types of bones.

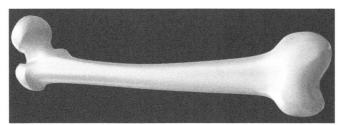

Long bone
(femur or thighbone)

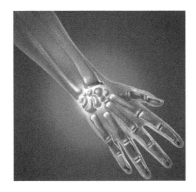

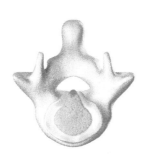

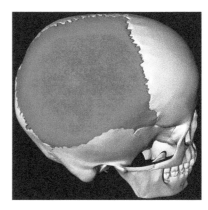

Short bone
(carpal or wrist bone)

Irregular bone
(vertebral bone)

Flat bone
(parietal bone from
roof of skull)

FIGURE 4–4. Examples of bones of different shape categories.

© dream designs, 2013. Used under license from Shutterstock, Inc. © Lightspring, 2013. Used under license from Shutterstock, Inc. © JCELv, 2013. Used under license from Shutterstock, Inc. © CLIPAREA, 2013. Used under license from Shutterstock, Inc.

Activity 4–2.   Locate the bones in the Figure 4–4 on yourself or a partner. Can you name and locate at least one other bone of each type?

Bones are mainly composed of minerals, water and protein. The minerals (mainly calcium and phosphorus) provide structure and strength while the protein, primarily in the form of collagen, provides resilience and keeps the bones from being too brittle. While we typically think of bones as static structures, they are not inert objects. Rather, they are living, cycling, tissues. They have blood and nerve supplies and have areas of formation and resorption. For the first 16–20 years of life, the bones grow. Most of the bones we will study in exercise science are referred to as endochondral, and develop from a cartilage base. As the long bones mature or calcify, they retain an epiphyseal growth plate at each end. When this growth plate fully calcifies or "closes," the bone stops growing in length. However, even though the length of a bone stops growing at around age 16–20, growth in diameter (or decreases in diameter) can continue, as the material in a bone will be broken down and replaced many times in a person's life. Osteoblasts and osteoclasts are cells responsible for the formation and resorption of bone, respectively. This formation and resorption of bone generally occurs in response to loads placed on the bones. This response is known as Wolff's Law, which states that bone will form in areas of stress and resorb in areas of disuse—"use it or lose it." Most people lose bone tissue as they age past about 45 years in women and 65 years in men. This is referred to as osteopenia, and in extreme cases the loss of bone leads to osteoporosis, which is a critically low bone mineral density and often results in fractures, particularly of the hip and spine. Growth and remodeling of bone is covered in greater depth in classes such as Anatomy and Physiology.

Joints and Joint Structure

Bones have what we call landmarks on them. Three of these landmarks are fossas, condyles, and tuberosities (see Figure 4–5). A fossa is a depressed (concave) area on the bone, while a condyle is a rounded (convex) spot, often on or near the end of the bone. These two areas on adjacent bones typically articulate (fit together) to form a joint. A tuberosity is a raised area where a ligament or tendon can attach.

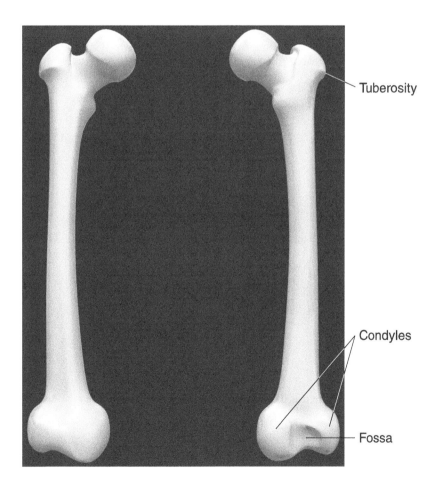

FIGURE 4–5. Diagram of a femur with fossa, condyles and tuberosity labeled.

© dream designs, 2013. Used under license from Shutterstock, Inc.

A joint is simply defined as the point(s) of articulation between two or more bones. There are numerous types of joints, which are distinguished by the amount and type of movement within the joint (Figure 4–6). Most sources define three categories of joints:

Synarthrodial: these joints are immovable by design. The joints of the skull, for example between the frontal and parietal bones, are synarthrodial "suture" joints. The joint between a tooth and the jaw bone (mandible and maxilla) is also a synarthrodial joint. If your teeth move in their sockets it is not generally a good sign except during childhood when you lose your first tooth. Since no movement occurs, synarthrodial joints may be described as nonaxial joints in older texts.

Amphiarthrodial: these joints provide a very slight degree of movement, but are not designed to be highly mobile. A symphysis, such as the pubic symphysis is an example of this type of joint. Intervertebral articulations (one vertebra to the next) are also amphiarthrodial joints.

Diarthrodial: these joints are freely movable. They are also known as synovial joints because of the synovial fluid which helps lubricate the joint. Within the broad classification of diarthrodial joints, there are usually described three subcategories with which you should become familiar, since these are the types of joints you will work with a great deal in clinical or exercise practices.

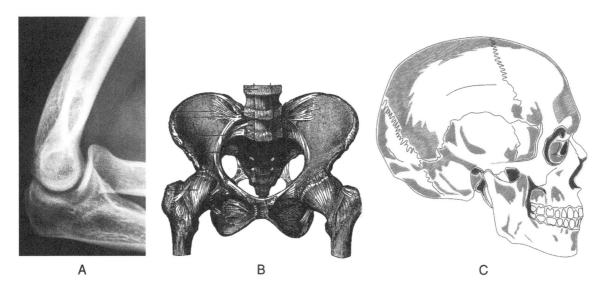

A   B   C

FIGURE 4–6. Examples of the three main categories of joint: diarthrodial the elbow (**A**), amphiarthrodial, the pubis (**B**), and synarthrodial, the skull (**C**).

Rather than focus on the names of the diarthrodial joint subtypes, it is instructive to focus on the degree of movement possible in each of the subtypes. Based on this criterion, the diarthrodial joints can be divided into three main categories. These are often referred to as uniaxial, biaxial, and multiaxial, because they allow movement in one, two or three planes, respectively (Figure 4–7).

The uniaxial joints are also referred to as hinge or ginglymus joints. The uniaxial joints allow motion in only one plane and consist of the knee and elbow. In a healthy elbow, can you move the joint any other way than open or closed?

Biaxial joints allow motion in two planes. An example of a biaxial joint is the wrist or radiocarpal joint. It can flex or extend, and it can adduct or abduct. If you try to move your wrist in any other manner, such as rotating, what happens to the radius and ulna (the long bones in the forearm)? They start to move, indicating that something other than the wrist joint is being moved.

The hip and shoulder are the two most common examples of the multiaxial joint. Notice how you can move your hip. It can be flexed, extended, abducted, adducted, and rotated. This may, in some cases, increase the likelihood of injury in this joint, for example the shoulders of swimmers are injured relatively often.

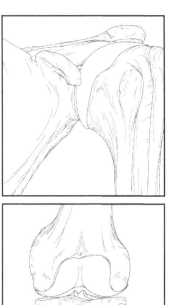

The shoulder, a multiaxial joint.

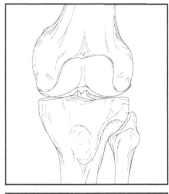

The knee, a uniaxial joint.

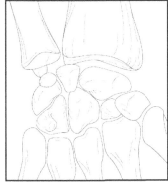

A biaxial joint, the wrist.

FIGURE 4–7. Examples of diarthrodial joints of different types and the planes in which they move.
© Kendall Hunt Publishing

Activity 4–3.   Locate and name at least one more uniaxial, biaxial and multiaxial joint on yourself.

The range of motion is a common consideration in the assessment of a joint. Range of motion (ROM) is the amount of movement a joint can make within a given plane without causing pain. The ROM is, in fact, a function of the joint itself. The normal movement of the joint is limited by its anatomy. For example, can you bend your elbow backwards more than a small amount? No, this is due to the structure of the joint. The ROM can also be affected by pathological problems like arthritis or bone spurs in the joint. These may anatomically limit the ROM by the damage they have done to the bone, or they may functionally limit motion because of pain. ROM may also be limited by the ligaments, tendons, and muscles surrounding the joints. We generally describe this effect as flexibility and it can often be improved by stretching exercises.

Tendons and Ligaments

Tendons and ligaments are structures that connect muscle to bone, and bone to bone, respectively. Both are made up of connective tissue, primarily collagen and elastin. In a muscle, there is connective tissue, mostly collagen, which surrounds each muscle fiber. At the end of the muscle, there are not any muscle fibers left, with only connective tissue remaining to form a tendon. In this way, it is an integral part of the muscle, but at the ends, where the attachment to bone occurs, only tendon remains. The characteristics of tendons make them very strong. This allows them to withstand high forces without stretching or tearing in most cases. They are also generally smaller in diameter than the muscles to which they are attached. This allows for the force from the muscle to pull on a tendon from a distance and still have an effect on a joint. The classic example of this action is in the hands. Look at the back of your hand, where only tendons occur. Now, use your muscles to hyperextend your fingers. Where is the muscle contracting? They are the muscles in the back of the forearm. Tendons, though, do not have as much blood flow as do muscles, or even bones. This means that if they are damaged, they take a long time to heal, and even when they do heal, they may not be as strong as before. Many times, tendons are surgically repaired using grafts from other parts of the body, or artificial grafts to make them stronger after the period of healing is over.

Ligaments have some similarities to tendon, but are somewhat more elastic. They have to have more stretch than tendons in order to allow the joint to move at all. In connecting two or more bones, they provide stability to the joint and help prevent it from moving in a way that would be harmful.

Muscles and Muscle Structure

There are literally hundreds of muscles in the human body. Experts disagree on the exact number, and the number may vary between people due to embryologic differences. When we discuss muscles in functional anatomy, we are generally talking about skeletal or striated muscle. Keep in mind that the heart is a muscle of a different type, and we have another type of muscle, smooth muscle, in areas such as the blood vessels, airways, and digestive system. Figure 4–8 shows the major skeletal muscles in the human body.

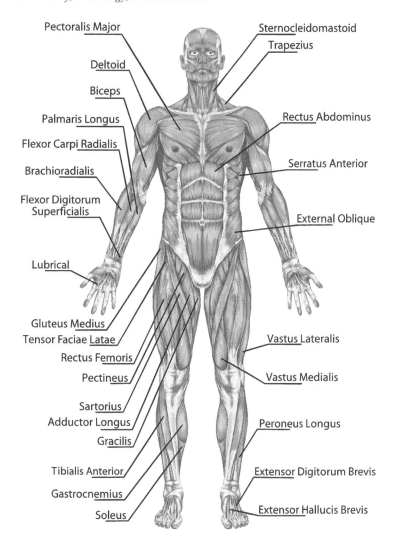

Pectoralis Major

Deltoid

Biceps

Palmaris Longus

Flexor Carpi Radialis

Brachioradialis

Flexor Digitorum
Superficialis

Lubrical

Gluteus Medius
Tensor Faciae Latae

Rectus Femoris

Pectineus

Sartorius
Adductor Longus

Gracilis

Tibialis Anterior

Gastrocnemius

Soleus

Sternocleidomastoid

Trapezius

Rectus Abdominus

Serratus Anterior

External Oblique

Vastus Lateralis

Vastus Medialis

Peroneus Longus

Extensor Digitorum Brevis

Extensor Hallucis Brevis

FIGURE 4–8. Diagram of the human skeletal muscle system.

© shitii, 2013. Used under license from Shutterstock, Inc.

Skeletal muscle physiology was already covered in Chapter 2, as you may recall. Each muscle is made up of myofibrils composed mainly of actin and myosin in a sarcomere structure. Although each individual sarcomere produces a similar force, different muscles, which are composed of millions of sarcomeres, can develop different amounts of force. One simple explanation for the different force capabilities of different muscles is the number of fibers, and correspondingly the number of sarcomeres. That is, more sarcomeres lead to a higher force production. It is also important to note, though, that different forces and speeds of contraction can be attained, even in muscles with similar fiber type make-ups.

Another reason for the differences in force generation is the shape of the muscle. In general, the more the muscle fibers are arranged in parallel (in the same direction), the greater the ability of that muscle to lengthen and shorten, often rapidly. The more the muscle fibers are arranged at an angle to their tendons, a structure known as pennate, the greater the cross sectional area and the greater the force produced, but the less the ability to lengthen and shorten. There are two main categories of muscle fiber arrangement, parallel and pennate.

Parallel muscles have all the fibers oriented along the axis of contraction. There are several subcategories of parallel muscle, including fusiform, flat and triangular, but in each case the fibers run parallel (or very nearly so) to one another. A classic example of a parallel muscle is the biceps brachii, or more commonly known simply as the biceps. Pennate muscles have a tendon running along the length of the muscle and the fibers are oriented at an angle to the tendon. A familiar object with a pennate structure is a bird feather. A bird feather has a central structure with fibers attached at an angle. If the muscle fibers insert on only one side, the muscle is termed unipennate. If the fibers are arranged along both sides, the muscle is called bipennate. If there are several tendons with the fibers running at an angle between them, this is termed multipennate. The greater force capacity of the pennate muscle comes with a cost, less ability to lengthen and shorten. The contraction of each fiber pulls on the central structure (tendon) at an angle, meaning that the force is applied both parallel and perpendicular to the orientation of the muscle, so less is applied directly in the line of the pull, and less shortening takes place. See Figure 4–9 for diagrams of the primary muscle arrangements.

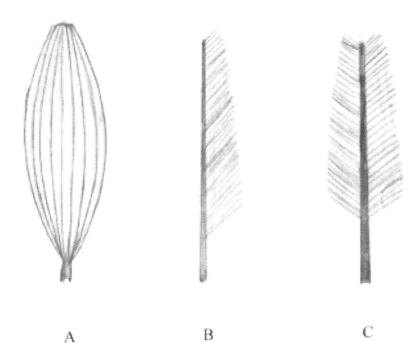

A   B   C

FIGURE 4-9. Diagram of muscle fiber arrangements: parallel (**A**), pennate (**B**) and bipennate (**C**).

Activity 4–4.   Why would a parallel muscle be able to shorten farther than a pennate muscle? Try drawing a parallel muscle and a bipennate muscle of the same size and see for yourself (hint: you will need to draw in the fibers as they would appear also).

Biomechanics

Biomechanics is the study of the forces and motions in living systems. It involves the application of mathematics and physics to motion. There are two areas of biomechanics, statics, and dynamics. Statics refers to the study of the system when it is constant, either at rest (not moving), or moving at a constant velocity and direction. Dynamics is the study of the system when it is accelerating, decelerating, or changing direction.

Biomechanics is also broken down into two other categories, kinematics and kinetics. Kinematics deals with describing a motion in terms of time and space. We might describe the displacement of an object or the distance it has travelled. These sound like the same thing, but are not. Displacement is the linear distance between an object's starting and ending points, while distance is how far the object has moved in getting from its starting to its ending points. Likewise, we also draw a distinction between velocity speed. Velocity is the displacement divided by the time it took the object to move, while speed is the distance divided by the travel time. The differences between these can be seen when running around a 400m track. If you complete one lap, the distance you have traveled is 400m, but if you start and finish at the same place, your displacement would be zero. If it took you two minutes to run the lap, your speed would be 400m/2min, or 200m/min, while your velocity would be 0m/2min, or 0m/min. Acceleration is the change in velocity over time. Acceleration can be positive or negative. We describe a negative acceleration as deceleration. Acceleration requires that a force acts on a body. This force can be internal, such as muscle activity, or external, such as gravity or friction acting to speed up or slow down the object.

Kinetics focuses on the forces that accompany a movement. For example, how much force is needed to jump one foot in the air? Or how much force would be needed to stop a car travelling at 50 mph? As these examples imply, force is related to the mass of the object as well as to its acceleration or deceleration. The higher the mass, or the quicker we want to accelerate or decelerate it, the more force is needed. Specifically, force is the produce to these two parameters, or:

Force = Mass X Acceleration

It is measured in pounds or Newtons (N). One pound equals 4.45 N. Please remember that while force and mass are related, they are not the same thing. A confusing concept for many students is the difference between weight and mass. Weight is the force our body exerts due to gravity, while mass is the amount of "stuff" or matter that makes up the object. If we change gravity, like on the moon (about 1/6 the gravity of earth), our weight will be decreased, but the mass will be the same as it is here on earth.

These aspects of biomechanics are important in analyzing the movements seen in sports, such as throwing a discus. Questions such as how fast the thrower's arm needs to be moving to get the disk the farthest, what is the optimum angle for release of the disk, and how much force is exerted by the thrower's legs during the throw can all be answered. They are also important in clinical situations, such as accidents. For example, biomechanists are involved in seat belt design, in the "crumple zones" of automobiles, and in analyzing what forces might have been required to cause a broken bone or damage to a tendon or ligament.

Stability and Center of Gravity

An object's center of gravity is the point where it is equally balanced in all directions. Theoretically, if you could find the center of gravity, you would be able to balance a body on a cane, like the Cat in the Hat. For symmetrical things, this is relatively easy. For a human, this is more difficult because we are not symmetrical—and we move! You have probably seen examples of some acrobats who balance well on very small things like a ball, rope, or another acrobat's hand. In order to do this, they have to have the center of gravity right over the pivot point made up by the ball, hand, or rope.

In addition to having the center of gravity above the pivot point, the acrobat has to be stable. Stability is the resistance to disruption of equilibrium of the body. Balance is the ability to control the stability. Many factors affect stability and balance. Among these are the mass of the body—the larger the mass, the greater its stability. The height of the object, particularly its center of gravity, affects stability. It is easier to tip over a tall object than a short one. Finally, the base of support is important in stability. In general the larger the base of support, the more stable an object. Let's look at a few examples. Keep in mind that a stable object is more resistant to movement than a non-stable object. In a football game, who is more likely to be moved, a 300 pound lineman, or a 160 pound kicker? (greater mass => greater stability). Is it easier to tip over a soda can or a hockey puck? (taller => less stability). Is it easier to push me over if I stand on one foot or on two feet spread shoulder width apart? (greater base of support => greater stability (Figure 4–10).

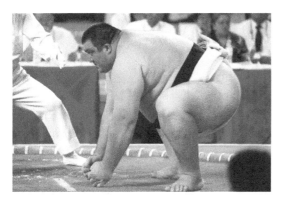 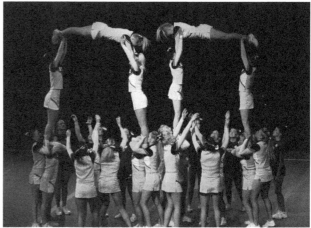

FIGURE 4–10. Which is more stable or less likely to be tipped over?

© testing, 2013. Used under license from Shutterstock, Inc.
© Aija Lehtonen, 2013. Used under license from Shutterstock, Inc.

Activity 4–5.   Working with a partner, try adjusting your height. For example, see if your partner can push you off balance easier in a standing or a kneeling position. What about with your feet together, or spread apart? What do these two exercises illustrate about stability?

Stability and center of gravity are not only important for when one is not moving, but help us perform many activities. Notice what happens when you turn on a bicycle. In order to turn, you have to lean into the turn. This is more apparent the faster you go. For example, watch road racing motorcyclists and notice how far they lean into a corner. What would happen if they didn't lean as far? This activity performs two functions, it helps keep your center of gravity within the area encompassed by the circle of the turn, which improves stability. It also lowers the center of gravity, again increasing stability.

Newton's Laws of Motion

Sir Isaac Newton worked in a number of areas, but one of the most famous is mechanics. He established three basic laws of mechanics which, if you understand them, make the understanding of biomechanics much easier.

Newton's first law is more commonly called the law of inertia. It states that a body at rest will remain at rest unless acted upon by an external force. Further, a body at a constant velocity will remain at that velocity unless acted upon by an external force that changes its velocity or direction. What happens if you lay a book on the ground? Does it move? No, the book has inertia and a force needs to act on it to make it move. If you push it or lift it and caused it to move, you have placed a force on it greater than its inertia. But if you throw a ball it will eventually slow down and stop. Why? Even though you may not see them specifically, there are forces acting on that ball. Air resistance may slow it down, and gravity causes it to fall to the ground. Then, rolling resistance acts as a further force to slow it down.

Newton's second law of motion is known as the law of acceleration. This law says that an object's velocity will change in magnitude (accelerate or decelerate) in direct proportion to the force acting on it and inversely in relation to the object's mass. If you throw a ball, you can throw it fast or slow, in relation to the force you put on it with your arm. Alternatively, how fast can you throw a baseball compared to a medicine ball?

Newton's third law is known as the law of reaction. It states that for every action, there is an equal and opposite reaction. More simply stated, if I exert a force on an object, such as holding a book in the air, that book is also exerting a force on me. My force is in the upward direction, while the book, acting with gravity exerts its force in the downward direction.

Types of Motion

Now that we know the laws of mechanics or motion, it is appropriate to define and describe the forms of motion that we undergo when we apply these forces. The types of motion are generally classified as linear, angular and general (Figure 4–11). Linear motion is where all parts of the system, whether it is a person or an object, move in the same direction at the same velocity. This is sometimes referred to as translation, because the object or person is being translated from one place to the next. Linear motion can be subdivided into rectilinear and curvilinear motion. A bicyclist coasting on a level road undergoes rectilinear motion since he is not pedaling and all parts of his body are moving in a straight line. A downhill skier in the tuck position who goes over a jump undergoes curvilinear motion. Notice that this person will stay in the tucked position, but will follow a curved line during his path from the take-off to the landing. Pure linear motion is not common in human activity.

Angular motion is movement around an axis. It is sometimes also referred to as rotation. Simply turning your head is an example of angular motion. The motion that a figure skater does by rotating very rapidly on her skates near the end of a routine is also an example of angular rotation. So, unlike linear motion, the whole body does not need to do the same thing. Angular motion is very common in human activity, since the rotation can occur at many joints, notice what happens at the hip or knee when walking or at the shoulder during a softball pitch. The force that causes the rotation is termed torque.

General motion is a combination of linear and angular motion. A person walking has her body translated from one place to the next as a result of angular motion of the joints of hip, knee, and ankle.

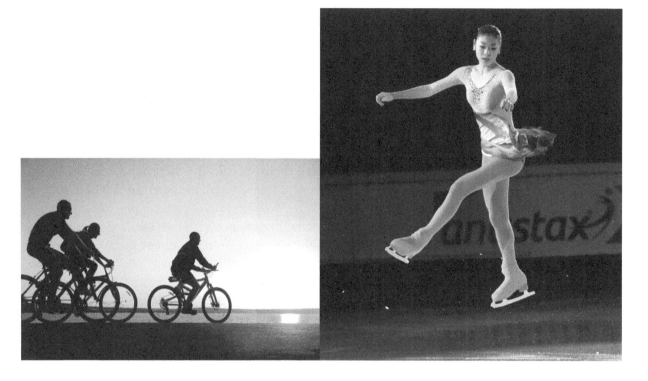

FIGURE 4–11. Diagrams of linear (bicyclist coasting) and angular (ice skater in an axel jump) motion.
© Yan Lev, 2013. Used under license from Shutterstock, Inc. © Diego Barbeieri, 2013. Used under license from Shutterstock, Inc.

Activity 4–6.   Climb the stairs in the room, or step up and down on your seat. What type of motion are you undergoing? Are any areas of your body undergoing a type of movement different from that of your whole body?

Classification of Levers within the Body

Now that you know about rotation and torque and have been through the concept of muscles and joints, it is useful to put that knowledge to use in understanding levers. A lever is one of the simple machines you learned about in grade school science class. A lever is a rigid structure attached to a fulcrum. The classic lever in the playground is the seesaw. The fulcrum acts as an axis and you use a force to move a resistance. There are different classifications of levers based on where the force, resistance and axis are compared to one another. In biomechanics, the fulcrum or axis is denoted "O," the force or effort to produce the motion is termed "E," and the resistance to movement around the axis is termed "R."

A first-class lever has the force and resistance on opposite sides of the axis—like a teeter-totter (see Figure 4–12). Some like to remember this as "EOR." As you can see, the fulcrum is between the force and the resistance. In the human body, the triceps muscle and the elbow act as a first class lever. Notice the insertion of the triceps muscle on one side of the elbow (at the end of the ulna) and the force is on the other side of the elbow—often at the hand.

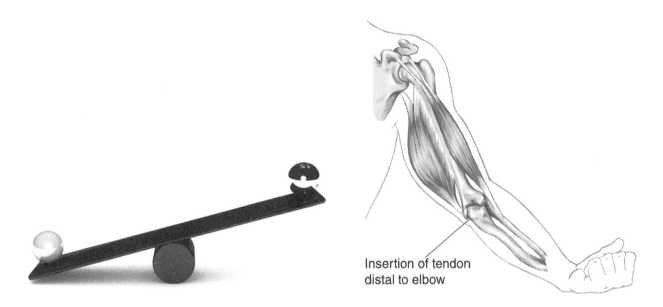

Insertion of tendon
distal to elbow

FIGURE 4–12. The seesaw and the combination of the triceps muscle and the elbow joint are examples of first class levers. Notice where the axis is in relation to the force and the resistance. Can you think of another example in the human body?

© 3DStyle, 2013. Used under license from Shutterstock, Inc. © shitii, 2013. Used under license from Shutterstock, Inc.

A second-class lever has the resistance placed between the fulcrum and the force. A good example of a second-class lever is a wheelbarrow (see Figure 4–13). Using the abbreviations above, the second-class lever is "ORE." The fulcrum is the wheel on the front, the effort is exerted by your hands and arms at the end of the handle, and the resistance is in the bed of the wheelbarrow. Second-class levers are rare in the human body. The brachioradialis muscle, an elbow flexor is an example. It inserts near the distal end of the radius bone, so the center of mass of the forearm (which is the resistance) is between the joint and the insertion of the muscle.

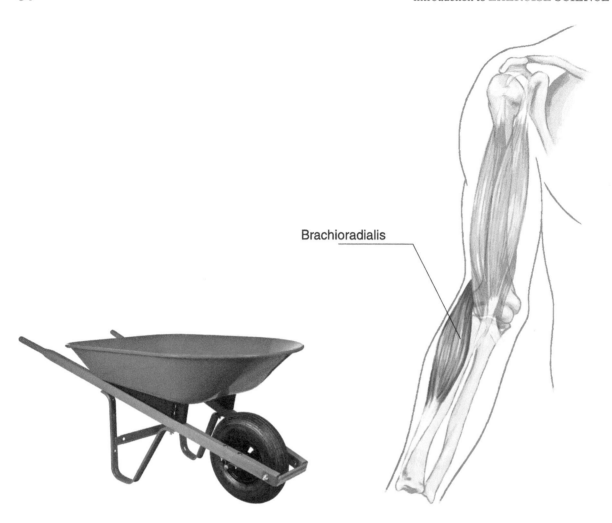

Brachioradialis

FIGURE 4–13. The wheelbarrow and the brachioradialis around the elbow are examples of second-class levers. Find the brachioradialis in yourself and see how it might work as a second-class lever.

© James Marvin Phelps, 2013. Used under license from Shutterstock, Inc. © shitii, 2013. Used under license from Shutterstock, Inc.

The third-class lever has the force placed between the fulcrum and the resistance. An example of this might be someone using an oar to row a boat. The hand held at the handle of the oar is the fulcrum, the hand pulling on the middle of the oar is the force, and the paddle in the water is the resistance (see Figure 4–14). The abbreviation for this type of lever is "OER." Many muscles in the human body are third-class levers. A good example of a third-class lever in the body is the biceps muscle in the arm. The fulcrum is the elbow joint, the force is the attachment of the biceps, and the resistance is the weight of the hand and anything in it.

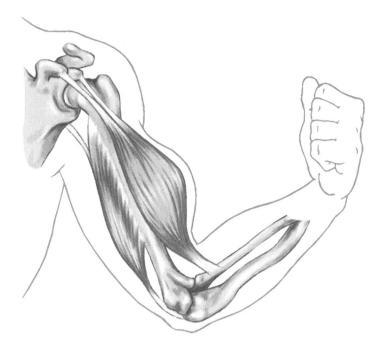

FIGURE 4-14. Diagram of the biceps muscle around the elbow, an example of a third-class lever. Notice the points of the fulcrum, force and resistance.

Mechanical Advantage

With the levers, there is another term called mechanical advantage. Mechanical advantage is:

Mechanical Advantage = Effort Moment Arm / Resistance Moment Arm

First, what is a moment arm? The moment arm is the distance from the axis of rotation at which the force is applied. As an example, go back to the seesaw example. If the seesaw is attached in the middle (where both moment arms are the same), the heavier object will always sink and lift the lighter object. If, however, the heavier object is moved far enough in toward the attachment (shortens the moment arm), the lighter object will lift the heavier object. See Figure 4–15 for this example.

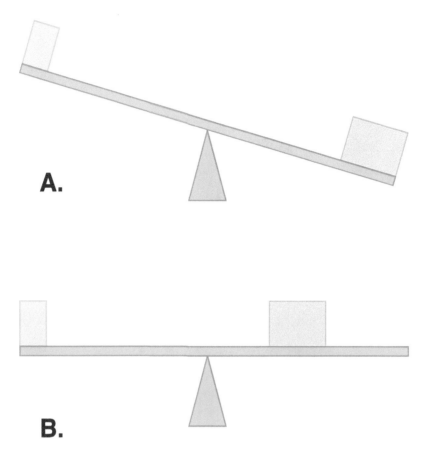

FIGURE 4-15. Diagram of seesaw with boxes at same distance from fulcrum (**A**) and with the heavier object moved inward (**B**).

So, the torque (rotational force) applied around the axis is directly related both to the force applied, and the length of the moment arm. Going back to the equation for mechanical advantage, you can see that if the effort (or force) moment arm is larger than the resistance moment arm, the mechanical advantage will be greater than one. The larger the mechanical advantage, the less force is needed to overcome the resistance and produce movement. Within the lever system, a first class lever can have a mechanical advantage either greater or less than one depending on where the axis of rotation is located in relation to the effort and resistance moment arms. How can this be? Go back—again—to the seesaw. If the side of the effort moment arm is longer than the other side, it will be a mechanical advantage greater than one. The opposite will be true if the side of the effort moment arm is shorter than the other side. A second class lever will always have a mechanical advantage greater than one. Keep in mind the wheelbarrow. The effort moment arm would be the handle and it is farther from the axis of rotation (the wheel) than is the load. A third class lever will always have a mechanical advantage less than one. To picture this, look at your forearm and biceps muscle. The muscle attachment (effort moment arm) is quite close to the elbow, while the resistance moment arm is the load in your hand.

Having a high or low mechanical advantage should not be associated with being good, bad, better, or worse, though, as other things are in play here. Mechanical advantage is generally in-versely related to speed or velocity. If you look at the third class lever, such as the biceps muscle as an example: The resistance torque is located farther from the axis of rotation than the effort torque. Since it is farther away from the axis of rotation, it travels further in the same period of time as the effort torque. A greater distance in the same time is a higher velocity. This is an advantage for throwing objects. Another example is the trebuchet, similar to a catapult, which is a first class lever. If we put a very large weight on one end with a short moment arm, and a long arm on the opposite end with a relatively small weight, that weight can be thrown a long distance (see Figure 4–16).

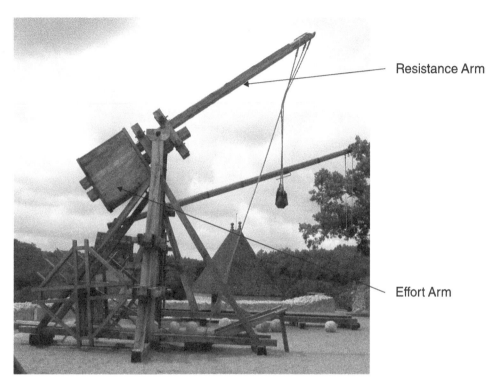

Resistance Arm

Effort Arm

FIGURE 4-16. Diagram of a catapult with the effort and resistance arms are noted. See how much shorter the effort arm is compared to the resistance arm.

© Laguii, 2013. Used under license from Shutterstock, Inc.

Loading

Now that we have covered the forces and actions involved in linear and angular movement, we can discuss forces that may or may not cause movements. These are termed loads. These forces can come from muscles, gravity, or other externally. There are three main types of loads, compression, tension, and shear (Figure 4–17).

Compression is a force that squeezes on the material. Think of it as if you placed a weight on top of a sponge. What would happen to the sponge? It is squeezed, or compressed. We see this in the spinal column of standing humans. The vertebrae are compressed by the ones on top of them.

Tension is the opposite of compression, essentially stretching or pulling. If you climb a rope in the gym, you are applying a tensile force, or tension, on the rope. In the body, we see tension applied by the muscles on the tendons attached to the bones, as the muscles contract.

Shear forces are applied in directions different from the long axis of the muscle or bone, but sideways or diagonally. If you apply a shear force on an object, you will get it to slide (or try to slide) along another object. By pushing a book along a desktop, you are applying a shear force to the book.

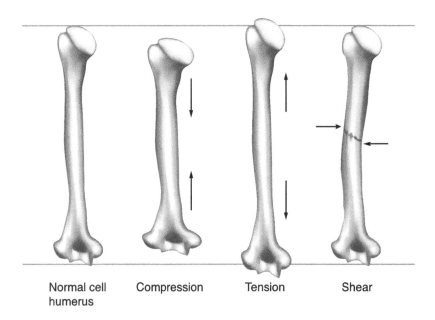

Normal cell   Compression   Tension   Shear
humerus

FIGURE 4–17. Diagram of the three types of loads, compression, tension, and shear.
© Kendall Hunt Publishing

Any of these forces can be either positive or negative. Loading a bone causes adaptations in that bone to increase its mass to withstand the forces applied. It has been shown numerous times that bone that is loaded will have a greater density. For example, the dominant arms of many tennis and volleyball players have a higher bone density than does the non-dominant arm (Calbet, 1999; Sanchez-Moysi, 2010). Excessive loading, though, can result in damage, such as fractures.

Areas of Study and Careers using Biomechanics

Biomechanics is most often divided into clinical and sport or exercise biomechanics. Clinical biomechanists use mechanical principles to analyze the occurrence and prevention of injuries, as well as to focus on treatment of those injuries. By evaluating the range of movement, the forces able to be generated by the patient and their deviations from normal, they can often point to a site that may have been injured or grown differently from the typical. Physical therapists often employ the principles of biomechanics, but the area of clinical biomechanics is growing with the aging of the population. Many people work in the areas of rehabilitation and in designing appropriate work and living spaces for older and disabled people, who need extra help in their environments.

Sports biomechanists concentrate on improving the performance in athletes. In addition, the sport biomechanist will work to prevent injury in the athletes. They evaluate the techniques of athletes and work to improve them so that the athlete can attain more speed or power during the activity, or do the activity in a way that requires less injury. Today, virtually every high jumper uses the technique in which they go over the bar backwards, leading with one arm and the head, with the back nearest the bar. Prior to the winning jump of Dick Fosbury in the 1968 Olympics, almost all jumpers used a rolling. It has been shown that the newer technique allows the athlete to raise his center of gravity higher earlier to clear the bar.

Another area in which biomechanics is often used is that of ergonomics. Ergonomics is the study of how humans and workplaces interact. Ergonomics experts perform many tasks designed to increase the productivity of workers and decrease the likelihood of injury in the workplace, either chronic due to repetitive strain, or acute due to overloading or accidents. An example of ergonomics in action is the office chair. There are many designs of chair that have come into common usage in just the last ten to fifteen years, with the goal of decreasing low back pain and neck strain on the job.

Glossary

Abduction—movement away from the body laterally.

Adduction—movement toward the body laterally.

Amphiarthrodial Joint—type of joint connection with limited movement, (e.g., vertebrae).

Anatomical Position—standard body position with arms to the side and palms forward.

Angular Motion—motion around an axis, also termed rotation.

Anterior—toward the front of the body.

Biaxial Joint—type of moveable joint in which the joint moves in two planes.

Center of Gravity—the point where the body is equally balanced in all directions.

Compression—forces acting to push on or shorten a body.

Condyle—convex or rounded area on a bone, often at a joint attachment.

Diarthrodial Joint—type of joint that is easily moveable.

Dynamics—part of biomechanics that deals with motion and changes in motion.

Extension—movement that involves opening or straightening a joint.

Flexion—movement that involves closing a joint or bending.

Fossa—concave or depressed area on a bone, often at a joint attachment.

Frontal—one of the cardinal planes that divides a body into anterior and posterior halves.

Fusiform Muscle—type of muscle formation in which all fibers are parallel along the longitudinal axis.

General Motion—type of motion that includes both linear and angular motion.

Hyperextension—movement that involves backward bending, opposition of flexion.

Inferior—toward the lower half of the body.

Kinematics—part of biomechanics that deals with describing movement.

Kinetics—part of biomechanics that deals with the forces that cause movement.

Lateral—toward the side of the body.

Linear Motion—type of movement where all parts of the body are moving in the same direction at the same rate.

Medial—toward the middle of the body.

Multiaxial Joint—type of diarthrodial joint that allows movement in all three planes.

Osteoblast—cell within a bone that causes bone to grow or increase.

Osteoclast—cell within a bone that causes bone resorption or destruction.

Pennate Muscle—muscle formation in which fibers are arranged at an angle from a tendon that is situated along the main axis of the muscle.

Posterior—toward the back half of the body.

Range of Motion—the amount movement a joint can undergo without causing pain.

Rotation—angular movement in the transverse or horizontal plane.

Sagittal—one of the cardinal planes of the body that divides the body into right and left halves.

Shear—forces acting on a body in opposite directions at different parts of the body.

Stability—resistance to disruption of a body.

Statics—part of biomechanics that deal with a body that is either not moving or if moving is not changing direction or speed.

Superior—toward the upper half of the body.

Synarthrodial Joint—a type of joint that does not move, by design.

Tension—forces that tend to pull on or lengthen a body.

Translation—another term for linear motion.

Transverse—a cardinal plane of the body that divides it into upper and lower halves.

Tuberosity—a formation on bone to which a tendon or ligament attaches.

Uniaxial joint—a type of joint that moves in only one plane.

References

General References

Floyd, R. T. 2009. *Manual of Structural Kinesiology*, 17th ed. New York: McGraw Hill.

Hall, S. J. 2012. *Basic Biomechanics*, 6th ed. New York: McGraw Hill.

McGinnis, P. M. 2005. *Biomechanics of Sport and Exercise*, 2nd ed. Champaign, IL: Human Kinetics.

Potteiger, J. A. 2011. *ACSM's Introduction to Exercise Science*. Philadelphia: Wolters Kluwer/ Lippincott, Williams and Wilkins.

References to Specific Studies

Calbet, J. A., P. Dias Herrera, and L. P. Rodriquez. 1999. "High Bone Mineral Density in Male Elite Professional Volleyball Players." *Osteoporosis Int.* 10:468–74.

Dietz, 2003. V. "Spinal Cord Pattern Generators for Locomotion." *Clin Neurophysiol.* 114:1379–89.

Nandi, D., T. Z. Aziz, X. Liu, and J. F. Stein. 2002. "Brainstem Motor Loops in the Control of Movement." *Mov. Disord.* 17 (Suppl 3):S22–S27.

Sanchis-Moysi, J., C. Dorado, H. Olmedillas, J. A. Serrano-Sanchez, and J. A. Calbet. 2010. "Bone and Lean Mass Inter-arm Asymmetries in Young Male Tennis Players Depend on Training Frequency." *Eur J Appl Physiol.* 110:83–90.

Chapter 5

MOTOR CONTROL, LEARNING, AND DEVELOPMENT

The global term **motor behavior** includes the three disciplines of **motor control**, **motor learning**, and **motor development**. These disciplines are sometimes separated and sometimes linked. In general, motor control refers to the neurological processes that result in movement. Motor learning encompasses how we learn new movements, including how different practice schedules and teaching techniques can help or hinder learning. Traditionally, motor development was the term applied to how we learn new tasks as we grow from infancy to adulthood, but now it is also used when we discuss the regression that takes place as we move from adulthood to old age, and the means by which we accommodate to the loss of visual acuity, muscular strength, endurance and other variables that change as we age. It is easy to see how motor control, learning and development are all intertwined, and why they will be grouped in this chapter.

Concepts in motor behavior are used extensively in both athletic situations and in the area of rehabilitation. Keep in mind that the *physiological* adaptations to training are only part of improving performance of physical tasks. How many strong people do you know who may not be very good at the shot put? How many fast people do you know who are not skilled basketball or football players? What different techniques might you employ in helping an athlete run faster as opposed to helping a stroke victim walk again? There are important differences between simply training a physiological system and training for a specific skill, and these differences are part of what motor learning, control, and development are about.

Motor Control

Although skeletal muscles do the heavy lifting (sometimes literally) of movement, they do not control movement. Control is the role of the nerves. Nerves not only stimulate the muscles to initiate the contractions necessary for movement, but they also sense force and speed during movement, as well as have responsibility for coordinating movements in relation to the environment; such that, for example, you don't fall down if there is a change in running surface. The role of the nervous system in motor control, and thus also in motor learning and motor development, cannot be overestimated.

The Nervous System

The nervous system is divided into two major parts, the central nervous system and the peripheral nervous system. The central nervous system consists of the brain and the spinal cord, while the peripheral nervous system consists of all the nerves that innervate the rest of the body.

The central nervous system has the primary responsibility for processing sensory information and sending out commands to the periphery. Within the brain, there are several regions that have different responsibilities. The cerebrum is the largest portion of the brain, totaling about 80% of the volume. It is divided into five regions, or "lobes" (Figure 5–1). The outermost 3 mm of the cerebrum is called the cerebral cortex. In anatomy, "cortex" always refers to the outer area of a structure. Voluntary movements are thought to be initiated in the motor cortex, a specific region in the frontal lobe. The motor cortex has been mapped via brain stimulation studies of both dogs and humans. The iconic map is called a "homunculus" or "little man". A key feature of the motor cortex is that the area allocated to a particular part of the body is proportional not to the anatomical size of the body part, but rather to the capacity of that part of the body for fine motor control. So, e.g., the tongue, which must be controlled very specifically for swallowing and speech, is mapped to a large area on the motor cortex. A comparable sensory cortex is located in the parietal lobe. Within the area of exercise, its largest responsibility is initiating voluntary movement. When we make the decision to swing a bat at an oncoming ball or start running, that is a cerebral function. The cerebellum receives a great deal of the afferent input from the periphery that allows us to determine the type of movement we are making "on the fly." That is, the cerebellum acts as an integrator. It is very important in movements that rely on quickness, where voluntary actions might be too slow. An example of this is the reactions we make while jogging on an uneven surface. When the foot sets down on a rock, we notice it consciously, but we also adapt muscle contractions to prevent falling or losing balance during that step. The brainstem is the junction between the brain and the spinal cord, but serves purposes much more important than simply as a bridge. It consists of the medulla, pons and midbrain. The medulla is vitally important in control of the heart and ventilation. The pons also has responsibilities in ventilation and receives input from the periphery to that effect. Both of these structures also have effects on things such as posture and basal movement. Some new research has linked tremor disorders such as Parkinson's disease with the brainstem and stimulation of certain parts of this area may decrease tremors (Nandi, et al, 2002).

The spinal cord consists of nerves (groups of neurons) that travel from the brainstem through the vertebral column to exit at various levels in the back. The spinal cord contains both myelinated and unmyelinated neurons. Myelin is a fatty tissue that surrounds and insulates the nerve. Its primary purpose is to speed up conduction. Nerves with myelin can transmit action potentials as fast as 60m/sec, while unmyelinated neurons may be as slow as 1–2 m/sec. In general, the fastest nerves are the ones that control movement, such as the nerves that go to the legs, while the slowest nerves are the ones that respond to stimuli like pain. This may seem wrong, but if you think of the longest nerve as only about one meter in length, sensing pain within one half-second of when it occurs is not a real issue, but controlling movement while running needs to be really rapid. Disruption of the nerves in the spinal cord can cause paralysis. This is seen in trauma situations where the person has a "broken back," as well as certain diseases, such as poliomyelitis, usually simply called polio.

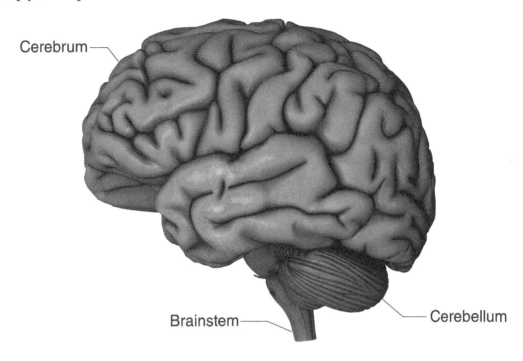

FIGURE 5–1. The human brain and its major portions: cerebrum, brainstem, and cerebellum.
© Anatomical Design, 2013. Used under license from Shutterstock, Inc.

The spine is important both as a conduit for neural inputs, or a "neural highway" from the periphery to the brain, and for the ability to perform some movements without the need for higher brain centers. These spinally-mediated movements are referred to as spinal reflexes. A spinal reflex involves input from one muscle or group and an output to that muscle (and possibly others). One of the simplest reflexes is the patellar or "knee jerk" reflex. When you lightly tap your patellar tendon with a rubber hammer or the side of your hand, the lower leg extends or "jerks." This involves a nerve carrying a message from the thigh muscles to the spinal cord, interfacing or synapsing with another nerve that goes back to that muscle and causing it to contract. This reflex involves only two nerves. This is also sometimes referred to as a reflex arc, an example of which is shown in Figure 5–2. Other spinal reflexes are more complex and can result in movements that look like locomotion in mammals such as cats. There is even evidence that there are "pattern generators" in the spinal cord that initiate movement at the spinal level. Spinal "pattern generators" are of keen interest to researchers attempting to help paraplegics walk (Dietz, 2003).

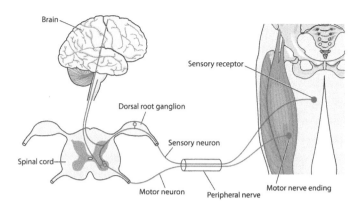

FIGURE 5-2. Diagram of the reflex arc.

© Blamb, 2013. Used under license from Shutterstock, Inc. © Alila Medical Images, 2013. Used under license from Shutterstock, Inc.

The peripheral nervous system consists of nerves outside of the brain and spinal cord. These nerves go to or innervate every area of the body. As in the spinal cord, there are both myelinated and unmyelinated nerves in the peripheral nervous system. This system is subdivided both by the direction the impulses travel and whether they are voluntary or not. Nerves that travel from the periphery, e.g., muscle, skin, eyes, ears, to the spinal cord are referred to as sensory or afferent neurons. These nerves take information *to* the central nervous system for processing. Those that go *from* the spinal cord to a muscle, sweat gland, or other organ, are called motor or efferent neurons. Within the motor neurons are two further subgroups. Those that we can control consciously are referred to as voluntary or somatic motor neurons. Good examples of these are the nerves going to the muscles of the arms or legs, which we can activate to move those limbs. The motor neurons that we cannot control voluntarily are termed autonomic. The autonomic neurons are further divided into sympathetic and parasympathetic groups. These control functions such as heart rate, the diameter of the blood vessels to regulate blood flow, and the activity of organs such as the stomach and intestines. See Table 5–1 for a description of the organization of the peripheral nervous system.

TABLE 5–1. Peripheral Nervous System Organization.

Category of Nerve?	Direction of Impulse Travel?	Also Known As?		Major Function(s)?
Afferent	Toward CNS	Sensory		Receive information from periphery within or outside of the body
Efferent	Away from the CNS	Motor		Send information to areas of the body
Somatic			Voluntary	Movement, speaking, eye movement
Autonomic			Involuntary	Heart rate, blood pressure, gut function

Particularly applicable to exercise and movement in general are a group of afferent neurons referred to as proprioceptors. Proprioceptors sense the amount and rate of shortening of muscles, the tension placed on a tendon and the rate and amount of movement of joints, among other things. The three main classes of proprioceptors we have that are important in movement are the muscle spindles, the Golgi tendon organs, and the joint receptors.

The muscle spindles are modified muscle fibers. They stretch more easily than normal muscle fibers and have sensory nerves attached. When the muscle spindle is stretched, the sensory nerve is activated and provides the brain information on how far the muscle is stretched and how fast. The knee jerk reflex discussed previously has muscle spindles as its sensory input. These spindles are stretched by a tap on the patellar tendon (simulating knee flexion), and respond by initiating a reflex causing the knee extensor muscles to contract. This proprioceptor is important in movement control, as it provides information both on the length of a muscle, indirectly showing the extension or flexion of a joint, and the rate of change of that length, which equates to the speed of movement.

The Golgi tendon organs are receptors in tendons that respond to the force exerted by the muscle attached to the tendon. Their response is to inhibit that muscle. This has been thought to be protective in that it prevents us from contracting the muscle so hard that we damage the tendon, which we already know is difficult to heal. It is also now known that this proprioceptor is important in control of movement. Since it is stimulated in relation to how hard the muscle is contracted, it helps us judge, both consciously and subconsciously, how hard we have to contract a muscle or group of muscles to get the desired force.

Joint receptors are a broad category of receptors located in the moveable joints. They respond to minor irregularities of the joint capsule to tell us how far open or closed a joint is and how fast it is opening and closing. Along with the muscle spindles and Golgi tendon organs, the joint receptor provide us with a tremendous amount of information about our movements, and provide feedback as to whether the movements we are doing are appropriate for our activity. Thus far, we have discussed how movements are controlled. The next step is to learn how we develop that control.

Motor Learning

Most of the time when we study motor learning, we do not focus on people who are already expert at a task, but rather on people acquiring the skill. For example, think about basketball players. If all you watch is someone who hits 80% of her free throws, all you see is a proper action for that person. What about someone who routinely hits 20% of free throws? You can watch the second individual to see mistakes that are made and how they can be corrected.

Prior to the 1970's, motor learning was generally thought of as a stimulus-response reaction. That is, when we are presented with a stimulus such as a visual cue or touch, we respond in a certain way. This model did not allow for explanations of how we vary our movements and react to very slightly different stimuli that might come about during an activity. This type of control is often referred to as task-oriented. Task-oriented control focuses on the effect of variables on the completion of a task or activity. Examples of this might be how far apart two objects are when the person is supposed to touch each in succession (see Figure 5–3). The farther apart, the longer it takes or the less accuracy there is with a task. Another example is the difference between a golf putt and a drive. We expect much greater accuracy with a five-foot putt than a 200-yard drive.

FIGURE 5–3. If you were asked move your hand at the same speed in both cases and to touch the two dots in **A**, or **B**, which would you most likely to be able to touch more accurately? This is an example of how the environment alters our ability to execute an accurate movement.

In the 1970's, the idea of process-oriented movement became much more prominent. The process-oriented approach takes into account how we assimilate stimuli and use different movement patterns to accomplish a task. The proponents of process-orientation argued that humans process information about how movements are viewed by the human and how they are stored in memory. It also uses errors while learning the movement to help process the information about the movement. This is an important consideration, as it takes into account feedback from misses to help us improve subsequent attempts. Using the above example in Figure 5–3, a process-oriented approach would have the subject watch the attempt (and its error) and feel the force and speed used by the hand moving between the two dots, integrate the two, and use that information to improve the next movement. We do this all the time, often without thinking about it.

Task and Environmental Dimensions

Think about all the possible movements you can do, from twiddling your thumbs to throwing a baseball pitch to running a marathon. Can you use common characteristics to group or categorize the movements? Motor behaviorists classify movements according to at least two schedules: discrete versus continuous movement and open versus closed movement. While classifications are always somewhat arbitrary, they help us remember both common and contrasting characteristics.

Figure 5–4 shows the relationship between discrete, serial, and continuous movements. A discrete movement is one which has a definable beginning and end, while a continuous movement has no beginning and end that can be recognized (at least not until the movement is stopped). Throwing a ball is an example of a discrete task. Taking a step is also an example of a discrete task. However, if you walk or run, you are taking multiple steps, that continue on and on, so this is a continuous task. Many researchers also use the term serial tasks within this classification. Serial tasks may take a prolonged time to complete, but are nonetheless one task. An example of a serial task is playing a piece on a piano. In this example, one has many discrete notes to play, sometimes even in repetition, but the end product is not simply the same note or string of notes put together. Instead it is many notes put together in a specific way. A serial task can be thought of as several (maybe many) discrete tasks put together. A key feature is that the *order* of the tasks is important. In a few minutes, virtually anyone can put together a succession of notes on a piano, but it takes someone with training to put them together in an organized (and pleasant) manner.

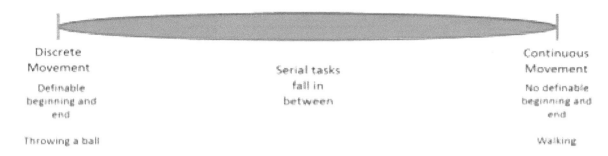

FIGURE 5-4. Schematic of discrete vs continuous movements (based on Schmidt and Lee, 1999)

Activity 5–1.   For each of these tasks, describe whether it is discrete or continuous—could it be serial? 1. Throwing a baseball; 2. Pitching a baseball game; 3. Tracking movements of an insect on the ground; 4. Steering a car along the highway; 5. Backing a car out of a parking spot.

A closed movement is one that takes place in an unchanging, or at least a predictably changing environment, while an open movement occurs in a constantly-changing environment that is often unpredictable. Batting while playing tee–ball, where the ball is set on a post and the batter hits it, is an example of a closed movement. In contrast, while batting against a good pitcher, who can throw at different speeds, at different spots around the plate and using different pitches, is an example of an open movement. Figure 5–5 shows the relationship between closed, mixed and open movements.

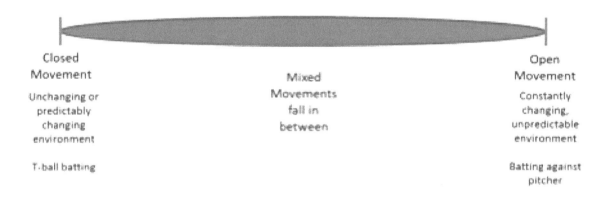

FIGURE 5-5. Schematic of open vs. closed movements (based on Schmidt and Lee, 1999)

Activity 5–2.   For each of these tasks, describe whether it is open or closed, or could it be mixed? 1. Catching a baseball from a pitching machine; 2. Catching a baseball hit in the outfield; 3. Catching a butterfly; 4. Catching an ant walking on the sidewalk.

Information Processing

Learning is not easy to define. What does it mean if you say you *learned* the material in this book? Does that imply you memorized the content, or more than that? If you know the content today, but have forgotten it in a month, have you really learned it? These questions are also relevant to motor learning.

A basic premise in the study of learning is that humans serve as information processors. That is, we get information from the environment, put it into our memory and process it. This processing can be simple (putting information into only one form of memory) or more multi-step, such as combining information or changing it from one form to another, like knowing the smell of something we see. Have you ever come across a skunk and backed away because you knew what a bad smell it can make? That is information processing. You recognized the skunk, associated one memory with another, chose a response, and executed it. In more general terms, information processing is often classified into three stages; a stimulus identification stage, a response selection stage, and a response programming stage. The stages can be viewed as seen in Figure 5–6.

Stimulus $\longrightarrow$ Stimulus Identification $\longrightarrow$ Response Selection $\longrightarrow$ Response Programming $\longrightarrow$ Movement

---

FIGURE 5-6. The stages of information processing. From the point of the stimulus to the point of the movement is often referred to as the reaction time, or RT.

The stimulus identification stage is when we take in or detect the stimulus and recognize it. This stimulus can be something visual (seen), auditory (heard), tactile (touched), olfactory (smelled), or a combination of these. This stage includes stimulus detection, where we actually take in the information and put it into a context that the brain can store. It also includes pattern recognition. Early in life, pattern recognition allows us to recognize the face of our mother or father (or other caregivers). Pattern recognition can also be much more complicated. A young chess master named Magnus Carlsen (www.cbsnews.com/video/watch/?id=7399370n) is able to play ten games of chess at once. Keep in mind that in chess, one has to see what the other player has done and has to plan ahead for future moves. Carlsen also did this without watching the boards! The ability to see what the board contains and to perceive what may lie ahead is inherent in the ability to become a good chess player.

The response selection stage of information processing follows stimulus identification. After a stimulus is identified, the person must decide what to do about it. Think about a goalie in soccer. In an uncharacteristically bad situation, the goalie may be faced with several offensive players from the opposing team and no defenders. The goalie sees the stimulus—a ball coming toward her accompanied by the opponents. She knows that one of the players is going to kick the ball toward the goal and she is likely to have only one attempt to stop it. So, she has to make a decision based on her knowledge of the situation and move in the direction she believes the ball is going to come from. This is her response selection. The speed and accuracy of response selection are affected by a number of variables. One of the primary variables is the number response alternatives. The greater the number of alternatives, the longer it takes to make a choice. Think how much more difficult the goalie's decision of where to expect the ball to come from will be if there are four offensive players than if there is only one player coming toward her with the ball. This is shown graphically in Figure 5–7.

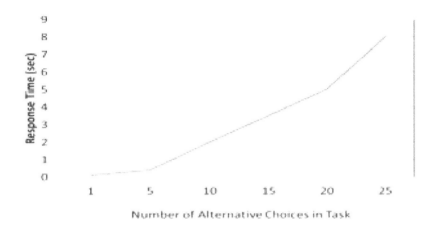

FIGURE 5–7. Relationship between number of response alternatives and the time it takes to make a choice.

The third stage of information processing is the response programming stage. By this time, the person has identified the stimulus and decided what the appropriate response is for the situation. Now the person has to perform a task. In the response programming stage, the person puts into action the response to the stimulus. The outcome of the response programming stage is the movement. The time taken for the entire process to occur is often referred to as the reaction time or RT.

If you examine an action like braking a car in an emergency situation we can break it down into the three stages, as in Figure 5–8.

Activity 5–3.   For each of the following activities, please break them down into steps using the stages of information model: Fielding a fly ball in the outfield; the goalie from the earlier example blocking an attempt on goal; swatting a mosquito on your arm.

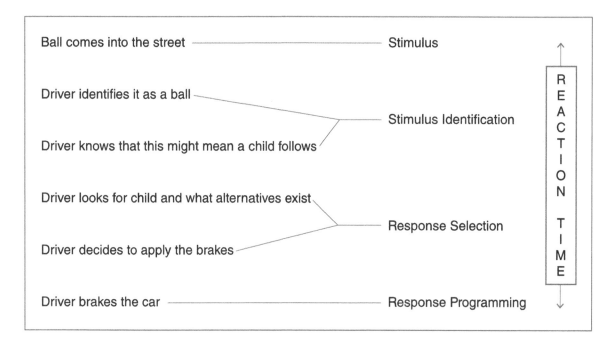

FIGURE 5–8. Stages of information processing in a real-life example.

Memory of Movements

While learning a movement, taking in the stimulus, processing it, and using that informa-tion to decide on and execute a movement is critically important in exercise, remembering that movement is also critical. Remembering movements and what they feel like when they are done correctly is a key part of learning. The predominant model to explain memory is the multistore memory model. This model suggests that as movements (as well as things like recognition of something like a face, or how to do a math problem) are being learned they are placed at different times in different types of memory or "stores." These types of memory include the short term memory store, short term memory, and long term memory.

The short term memory store is also sometimes known as the short term sensory store. It appears to be where large amounts of information are taken in quickly, but disappear quickly. An analogy might be the little bit of sound you hear for a second or so after you turn off a radio. The information is there initially, but goes away rapidly. The storage duration is thought to be less than one second, with a useful duration of only about ¼ of a second. The primary purpose of the short term memory store appears to be a way of taking in the information so that it can be en-coded and placed into one of the memory areas.

Short term memory is different from the short term memory store. The similarity in the term is unfortunate, but ingrained in the field, so continues to be used. It is sometimes called the working memory, because information in short term memory is thought to come from either the short term memory store, or from long term memory and is used soon. It has a relatively small capacity and relatively short duration, although not as short as the short term memory store. The capacity is generally thought to be around seven items, with duration no longer than 10–20 sec-onds (see Figure 5–9). Short term memory is also thought to involve "coding" or changing the image or memory into something abstract. In this way, we don't retain a number by its shape, for example, a 3, but we change the shape to the number three and store it that way, by a name, with a concept of its numerical value. Short term memory is also thought to relate to consciousness, or attention. If we haven't paid attention to the image it is not generally thought to get stored. In other words, we are aware of the things in our short term memory.

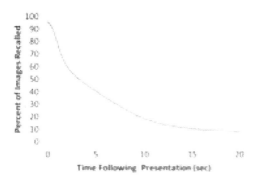

FIGURE 5–9. Relation of time to the recall of images.

Long term memory is the third category of memory. Items are placed in long term memory when they have been practiced a sufficient number of times. This gives us the ability to perform things that we learned previously, but have not done in a while. Watch a person who is a good athlete, but has been out of training for a while. The skills may not be as good as when she was in training, but are still better than the average person. This indicates that the person has remembered the skills used in the task, whether it is hitting a ball with a bat or throwing free throws. Can you remember your parents' address? This is another example of long term memory; it is something that you do not use all the time, but when you need to remember it, it is there. Another characteristic of long term memory is that it has a much greater capacity than short term memory. While short term memory is thought to have space for about seven items, long term memory has to be extremely large. Think of all the things you do in a day, from moving around to remembering the location of the bookstore or dining hall. All of these are stored in long term memory. Damage to the hippocampus (part of the brain) can decrease the ability to transfer information from short term memory to long term memory. What would this do to our ability to retain material?

Phases of Learning

When you watch someone attempt a new skill, you often notice "stages" in their development of that skill. That is, the person starts by having to think about every movement that is made, then improves upon those movements by relatively minor changes in movement pattern, and finally appears to have incorporated the movements into their basic knowledge or pattern. These phases of learning are termed cognitive, associative and autonomous, respectively.

During the cognitive phase, the person is new to the task and is trying to determine what is the best sequence of movements to accomplish the task. Generally the movements are slow and deliberate during this phase and improvements are rapid. Assistance in terms of feedback and instruction are often used during this phase. During the associative phase, subtle changes are made in the movements to improve the consistency and speed. During this phase, the improvements are more gradual and seem to rely more on the person's own perception of the movement, and less on outside coaching and instruction. This phase can last months, or even years. The autonomous phase is characterized by having the movement performed without outside coaching and often in the face of other things that might be distracting to someone at a less advanced stage of learning.

Let's take a rather complicated movement and go through the phases of it—typing on a keyboard. When first exposed to a computer keyboard, the tendency is to use the "hunt and peck" method. That is, we only use one or two fingers on each hand and we look for the location of each letter on the keyboard. If you are taking instruction in typing, the instructor might suggest where to put the fingers before starting. This lessens the amount of movement each finger has to make when finding a key, but we still look for every letter as we hit the key. During this time we get feedback from the computer screen, by the letter or number that appears, and we improve. This is definitely a cognitive phase, since we are thinking about each individual key we are tapping. As we improve, it is easier to let each different finger hit its own keys on the board and we are faster and make fewer and fewer mistakes as we progress. Many of us stay at this associative phase, but some get a lot of practice and move on. By the time we have practiced for quite a while, we are not only much faster, with fewer mistakes, but we can talk with peers, think about the movie we saw last night or many other things while still performing the task at a very high level. This is the autonomous phase and by this time we consider that we have mastered typing.

Learning vs Practice

While practice is likely to lead to learning, particularly if done correctly, practice and learning are not the same things. Learning indicates that there is a relatively permanent and consistent change in a skill level. Let's use the example of a golf putt. If you put the ball two feet from the hole and try to putt the ball in, you are likely to get better the more you putt. Eventually, you will be likely to make the large majority of the putts. However, if you move the ball to a different spot with a different slope or a longer distance, you will probably not do very well. How you structure practice affects learning, as we will see in the next section.

Factors Affecting Learning

As we just discussed, practice and learning are not the same things, but practice can affect learning. When we learn something, it becomes part of our skill set and something we can pick up later with a relatively high level of skill compared to before we learned it. These factors affect how we practice a task and how we set up practice for the people we are training, whether in a workplace or on an athletic team. What are the goals? The goals include being able to learn the task (acquisition), being able to remember the task (retention) and being able to use the task in other situations (transfer). These portions of learning are all evaluated in the transfer paradigm. In the transfer paradigm, the investigators measure the acquisition of the task, through something like the number of errors made, or the speed of the task. They then allow a period of time for rest/recovery, and later measure the performance of the task again. This is a measure of retention. While many factors can affect learning a task, the following sections cover some of the most important ones.

Number of skills learned at once

The greater the number of things that need to be learned at once, the less (or slower) will be the learning. This is referred to as contextual interference. While it is not simple to quantify, the concept is rather simple. If we think of being presented with a new task while we are learning one task, we can imagine that this will slow learning. In the golf putting example we used above, what would it do to your ability to learn to putt if someone gave you a longer or shorter putter every time you struck a ball? Here you not only have to learn the act of putting a golf ball into a hole, how hard to strike the ball and how to determine direction, but you are given a different club each time, which affects both how hard you hit the ball and how you pick the direction. From this example, you should be able to see that contextual interference should make learning a skill more difficult. Some argue, though, that while the acquisition of the task is lengthened, the retention of the learned task improves. The transferability of the task, or the ability to employ the learned task in different situations, may also improve.

Variability of practice

By varying the type of practice when a person is learning a skill, the acquisition appears to be poorer (takes longer to learn), but the retention seems to improve. This is somewhat similar to contextual interference, except the variability is within the same skill. If we think about shooting a jump shot in basketball, an invariable practice would have the person shoot from the same spot time after time, while practice variability has the person move around the basket to shoot from different distances and different angles. Variability of practice may be something that should be incorporated after the rudiments of the skill are mastered. For example, if you are trying to teach a 5-year-old to shoot a basketball, you first have to get him to the point where he has some idea of how hard to throw it to even get it to the basket and this may work better with invariable practice. But when the basics of the skill are mastered, introducing variable practice appears to be a better strategy for improving performance.

Feedback

If you do not get feedback on your performance you do not know whether you are doing the task correctly or not, so feedback is critical to learning a new skill. The study of feedback has been a major focus in motor learning for many years. Feedback is often abbreviated KR (knowledge of results) or KP (knowledge of performance). KR is information about the outcome of the movement. Examples of KR would be how many golf putts went in the hole out of ten shots, or the average distance the putts stopped from the hole. KP is information about the movement pattern or process. In the golf putting example, KP might include having someone tell you to bend over more, or to move the putter in a straight line. Feedback can be extrinsic (from outside). For example, did the ball go in the basket (visual feedback), a coach's or trainer's comments (verbal), or did the bat hit the ball (visual, auditory, touch). It can also be intrinsic (from inside). Simply asking yourself if the motion felt right is an example of intrinsic feedback. Feedback helps, but can be a crutch if we do not use enough sources. If you only use the feedback as to whether a golf ball went into the hole, you do not really know if you did the skill correctly or were simply lucky.

The way feedback is presented affects learning. We might think that feedback given after every attempt would help to improve learning, but quite the opposite seems to be true. Early in the learning of a skill, feedback given after every (or nearly every) attempt seems to help. For example, if you are practicing hitting a ball with a bat, having a coach show you how to do it, then tell you every time what you did correctly and incorrectly is probably helpful. After the basics of a skill are learned, though, feedback in a summary form seems to be more useful. Summary feedback can be given at a constant interval, such as every five attempts, or at a sliding interval, where early in learning it is given relatively often, but the interval increases with time. Generally, it appears that as the skill of the person doing the task increases, the amount of feedback needed decreases (Figure 5–10).

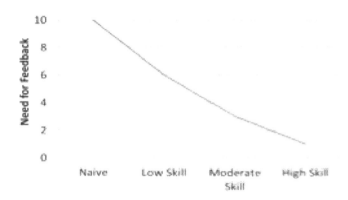

FIGURE 5–10. Relationship between skill level and need for extrinsic feedback.

Practice organization

If we organize our practice trials in different ways, we will get different results. Practice variability and contextual interference (from above) both decrease our performance during the practice itself, but appear to increase our learning. The ideal levels of variability and interference differ between people, but in general are dependent on the learner's skill and the difficulty of the skill. The higher the skill of the person and the higher the difficulty, the more variability and interference can be tolerated to improve learning.

When learning complicated skills such as swimming strokes, a discus throw, or a high jump, learning may be improved by at least two different strategies. These are the part-whole and the progressive practice strategies. The part-whole learning strategy takes a complicated movement and divides it into smaller parts that are easier to learn. For example, novice skaters do not learn a triple axel jump, but rather learn to perform one turn, then two, then advance to a triple. The progressive practice strategy would also work in figure skating. Using this strategy, the skater learns one type of jump, then another, then a spin, or whatever other skills are involved. Only when each of the skills are mastered, does the skater put them together into a routine. In real life, we often use both the part-whole and the progressive strategy for nearly every complicated skill.

Task difficulty and learning

Task difficulty is a general term for how hard a task is to learn. It can be related to the learner's experience. This is also called relative difficulty. For example, learning a new gymnastics routine will be much easier for someone with skills in gymnastics than a novice. Further, task difficulty can be related to the complexity of the skill. Learning to do a long jump properly is more difficult than learning to run down the runway to the take-off board. Finally, a task can be made more or less difficult based on the type and amount of feedback the learner receives. There are many examples of self-taught musicians, but it often takes them longer to learn than someone who takes lessons from a proficient teacher. There appears to be an optimal difficulty level for the greatest learning. This point is sometimes referred to as the challenge point. Below the challenge point, practice performance is high, but learning is low (again, think of practicing basketball shots always from the free throw line). Above the challenge point practice and learning performance diminish (think about practicing those free throw with Kobe Bryant challenging you). See Figure 5–11 for a graph of this effect.

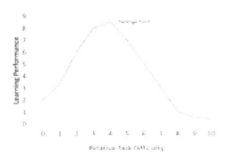

FIGURE 5–11. Learning graphed against the difficulty of the task.

So, as you can see, motor learning and control are complex fields with many variables. The goal is to teach skills to a performer, whether those are sport skills or work skills. Many organizations, from assembly lines to professional sports teams, hire consultants who are experts in motor learning to help their workers or athletes. These motor learning professionals use the knowledge of how we learn activities to increase productivity and decrease errors, and in doing so, help us become better athletes and workers who are less likely to get injured or injure someone else in performing our tasks.

Motor Development

Motor development is the study of the changes in motor behavior and exercise capabilities through the lifespan. The field has often been called growth and development because it concentrated almost exclusively on the process of motor behavior in children as they matured. It was a field very important to students studying physical education, who dealt with young people of different ages and it helped them know what skills and movements to expect students to be able to accomplish at different ages. This is still an important part of motor development, but the field has grown to increase its emphasis on adults and on the aging population. This change in the field has made it an important area of study for students desiring to enter clinical fields like medicine, physical and occupational therapy, where many work with children of different ages, but many deal with the adult population and the changes in their physical abilities as they age.

Theories Related to Development of Motor Skills in Children

During development, it is obvious that children and adolescents mature in both their abilities related to thought processes, as well as movements. There are a number of theories related to how children mature, and not all are mutually exclusive. The maturational theory, proposed by Ge-sell in the 1930's (Gesell, 1932), suggests that children develop based on genetic factors and that stimulation from the external environment (training) has little to do with this development. The idea behind this theory was that since the neural system had a genetic component to its develop-ment, the actions that babies and children learned would as well. This is the basis for many growth and development charts indicating when a baby should be able to roll over, crawl or walk, among other activities. This theory has been shown to be overly simplistic and it is now well known that environmental factors such as parental involvement and the presence of other children, among others, are important in development of motor skills.

The cognitive development, or intellectual development theory was developed by Jean Piaget in the 1930's, and only translated into English starting in the 1960's. Piaget suggested that the child interacts with his environment in a way that he seeks out information from the environ-ment. He also developed a scheme of stages of development. These are the sensorimotor (from zero to two years), the preoperational (from two to seven years), concrete operations (seven to eleven years) and formal operations (greater than eleven years). While these stages are not as broadly used as in the past, some still continue to use them. The importance of Piaget's work, even though some of it has been shown not to be correct, cannot be underemphasized, as he took a very scientific approach to childhood development that combined inherited and environmental parts.

More recently, several theories have been developed that try to encompass the things that happen during maturation that are genetic in nature and those that are more related to how we perceive and react to the environment around us. The environmental context theories, devel-oped by Bronfenbrenner (1986) and Gibson (1984), help provide a framework in which a child in-teracts with her environment to learn new tasks. Bronfenbrenner's ecological systems theory uses many different levels of environment that a child encounters to explain how they learn. These levels of environment include the microsystem, which is where the child lives. Here such things as family, peers and school play a role in her development. There is also the exosystem, in-cluding neighbors, mass media, and similar groups. The ecological perspective, proposed by the Gibsons, see a child as perceiving the world around her, which is sufficient experience to begin learning.

While none of these theories have been completely verified or debunked, it is increasingly obvious that learning among children is something that involves heredity, the environment, and interactions between the two. The different theories allow motor development researchers to study the learning of children and put the results of experiments into a cohesive process of how the child learns.

Stages of Development in Children

Regardless which of the theories concerning the maturation process is predominant, there is general agreement about stages of development. This helps students learning about motor devel-opment to place certain actions and skills into context, as to which should emerge at similar times. In general, the lifespan is characterized by stages of infancy, childhood, adolescence, and adulthood.

Infancy is the period from birth to approximately two years of age. Many movements can be performed, even early in infancy, but many of the early infancy movements are reflexive in nature. Primitive reflexes are usually for nourishment and protection. These include sucking and grasping. The sucking reflex is obviously related to nourishment and is initiated simply by touching the baby's face around the lips. This is a technique many young mothers learn to encourage a baby to nurse. The grasping reflex (Figure 5–12) is initiated by a touch to the palm of the baby's hand and is quite a strong reflex. Some photographs actually show babies grasping strong enough to be lifted off the ground while only holding on with one hand. A similar grasping reflex can be seen by touching the ball of the foot. When this is done, the toes of that foot curl under and a grasping motion, although obviously the ability to actually clasp an object will be much poorer with the feet than the hands. There are also several reflexes that appear to be at the root of locomotion that occur early in infancy. An example of this is the asymmetrical tonic neck reflex, in which if the head is turned to one side, the arm and leg on the side to which the head is turned extend. This is also called the fencing position reflex. These reflexes all occur very early in life, from birth to only 4–12 months. The persistence of some of these reflexes become warning signs of developmental abnormalities, but that is beyond the scope of this chapter.

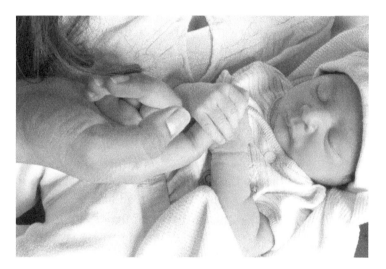

FIGURE 5–12. Grasping reflex in an infant.
© Tony Wear, 2013. Used under license from Shutterstock, Inc.

As infancy progresses, there are a number of motor skills achieved by children. These mainly involve improvements in locomotion and manual control. Some have called them landmarks and begin suspecting developmental abnormalities if they do not occur at specific times, while others believe it is just differences between children and do not start to become concerned about them unless the skills are greatly delayed. In locomotion, these landmarks consist of crawling, creeping, and walking. In crawling, the baby scoots along the floor using arms and legs but does not raise the stomach off the floor, while creeping is similar with the stomach clear of the floor. Walking also consists of several phases, including walking with and without support, and walking backward, which all usually occur during the first two years of life (Figure 5–13).

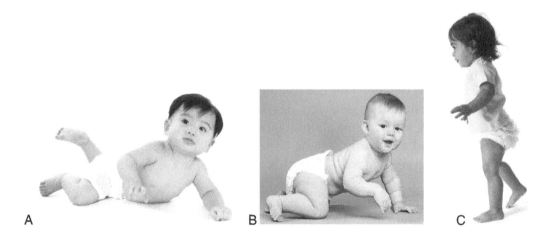

FIGURE 5–13. Examples of babies: **A.** crawling, **B.** creeping, and **C.** walking without support.
© iPortret, 2013. Used under license from Shutterstock, Inc. © Zdorov Kirill Vladimirovich, 2013. Used under license from Shutterstock, Inc. © picturepartners, 2013. Used under license from Shutterstock, Inc.

Childhood, the period from two to twelve years, is characterized by improvements in fundamental movements such as throwing, running and jumping. These activities are also referred to as movement patterns, and movement patterns can be classified as either immature or mature. An immature movement pattern means that the child can do the activity, while a mature movement patterns indicates proficiency at the pattern. When you have a chance, watch a child run. Little children use a more erect posture with their arms often out to the sides, and may not be able to maintain a straight line, while older children run more like adults, with a forward lean, arms to the sides and can usually run in a straight line.

Adolescence has not been studied to the same extent as childhood because many of the movements have been mastered at or near an adult level. With adolescence, one of the major changes seen is the differentiation between performances between males and females. There is a general leveling of skills in females, coinciding with the slowing of growth, while males still improve in many skills. We also see differences in strength and cardiorespiratory endurance beginning in adolescence which were minimal in childhood. Some of this difference may be sociological since historically girls were not encouraged to participate in high level sporting activities, but some are developmental and physiological, as we see differences in strength and cardiorespiratory endurance between men and women that are not related to differences in training.

Adulthood and Regression

Physical function is generally thought to peak somewhere around the age of 30. This is highly dependent on the person and his level of training through adulthood. This peaking is shown in numerous physiological measurements such as maximal oxygen consumption, strength and muscle endurance, as well as more cognitive measurements such as reaction and movement time. Most of the changes seen after the age of 30 seem to occur at the rate of about 10% per decade, or one percent per year (see Figure 5–14, for examples).

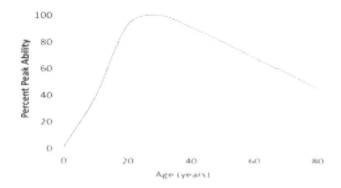

FIGURE 5–14. Relationship of many physiological parameters (e.g., Vo2max, strength, speed) with age.
Canadian Society for Exercise Physiology www.csep.ca

There are numerous theories for the decline in function with age. The genetic theory suggests that the human genome dictates the aging process. The theory suggests that the maximal human lifespan is approximately 125 years. Obviously, nobody lives that long, since the oldest recorded person was Jeanne Calment of France, who lived a remarkable 122.4 years, from February 1875, to August, 1997, but did not make it to 125 years. Therefore, there must be influences other than genetics that dictate aging. Various theories related to cellular mutations have been advanced to explain the aging process. These theories suggest that through metabolic processes, waste products are produced that lead to cellular mutations that lead to aging. Among these byproducts are free radicals or reactive oxygen species, which are produced as a result of aerobic metabolic processes. These have been shown to change the structure of various tissues, including blood vessels, possibly leading to death through heart disease. They have also been related to mutations leading to certain cancers, but the evidence for this is not yet conclusive. As we age, the immune system decreases its response, leading to a decreased ability to fight infections. We can see evidence for this in the increased rate of infectious diseases such as cold and flu in older people, and the increased death rate from these diseases in the elderly. While this doesn't explain aging itself, it does help explain why we do not reach the lifespan projected by the genetic theory.

Regression after age 30 can be modified with exercise. Several studies have shown that the declines in cardiorespiratory endurance can be cut in half (5% per decade) with even moderate exercise (Kasch, et al, 1999). Muscle strength also typically decreases at a rate of about one percent per year. As with cardiorespiratory endurance, the decline can be decreased. Sarcopenia, the loss of muscle tissue, though, seems to be accelerated later in life at a rate that exercise can keep up with. While it may seem contrary to a novice in the field, training can be highly effective in elderly subjects. Improvements in strength, aerobic capacity, and reaction time have all been shown with training. In the very elderly subjects, this may be something as simple as lifting a can of vegetables or walking with the aid of a cane or walker, or it can be a regular training program that might be applied to younger adults, but with appropriate modifications for safety and health issues.

Glossary

Acquisition—the process of learning a task.

Adolescence—stage of life from approximately 12–18 years. This is a period of rapid growth and maturation.

Adulthood—stage of life from approximately 18 years to the end of life.

Afferent—nerve that carries information to the central nervous system, often termed sensory.

Associative—phase in the learning process following cognitive. Improvements in this phase are more gradual and seem to rely on a person's own perception of the skill.

Autonomous—phase in the learning process following associative. Movements are performed without outside coaching and not affected greatly by distractions.

Brainstem—part of the brain that includes the medulla, pons and midbrain.

Cerebellum—part of the brain that acts as an integrator, particularly important for quick movements.

Cerebral Cortex—part of the brain that is primarily involved in voluntary movement and thinking.

Childhood—stage of life from approximately 2–12 years. This is a period of rapid improvements in movement skills.

Closed movement—a movement that takes place in an unchanging or predictably changing environment.

Cognitive—earliest phase in the learning process. Greatly relies on outside coaching and feedback.

Cognitive development theory—one of the hypotheses about aging and development in which a child interacts with his/her environment and seeks information from that environment.

Contextual interference—presentation of another task while we are learning one task. This appears to slow the learning of the task but improve the retention.

Continuous movement—a classification of activities that do not have a specific beginning or end, other than when we start or stop. Walking is an example.

Discrete movement—a classification of activities that have a specific beginning and end. Throwing a ball is an example.

Efferent—nerve that carries information away from the central nervous system, often termed motor.

Genetic theory of aging—suggests that the process of aging is programmed into our genome.

Golgi Tendon Organ—receptor in the tendon that senses tension.

Infancy—stage of life from birth to approximately two years. Many movements can be performed, but many early movements are reflexive in nature.

Joint Receptor—receptor in moveable joints that senses rate and amount of movement in the joint.

Knowledge of performance (KP)—feedback during the learning of a task that relies on information about the movement pattern. An example might be having a coach tell you to bend your knees more during the lineup prior to a football play.

Knowledge of results (KR)—feedback during the learning of a task that relies on information about the outcome of the activity. An example might be how many horseshoes landed within two feet of the post.

Long-term memory—part of the multistore memory model. Items go into long-term memory when they have been practiced sufficiently to be well known.

Maturational theory—one of the hypotheses about aging and development that suggests that development is based on genetic factors and that outside influences have little to do with it.

Motor behavior—field of study that includes motor control, motor development and motor learning.

Motor control—subdiscipline of motor behavior. This field deals with the neural processes that occur during the execution of a movement.

Motor development—subdiscipline of motor behavior. This area deals with the processes that occur in learning tasks as we develop and as we age.

Motor learning—subdiscipline of motor behavior which studies how we learn a new task and the processes that speed up and hinder that learning.

Muscle Spindle—receptor that senses length and change of length in muscles.

Myelin—lipid coating of a nerve that insulates and speeds up conduction.

Open movement—a movement that takes place in an environment that changes unpredictably.

Regression—the stage of development that deals with loss of abilities as we age during adulthood.

Retention—remembering a task after is has been learned.

Short-term memory—part of the multistore memory model, sometimes called working memory.

Short-term memory store—part of the multistore memory model. Large amounts of information are taken with the apparent purpose of placing it into one of the memory areas.

Summary feedback—information (KR or KP) about a movement that is presented at intervals as opposed to after each attempt.

Transfer—the ability to use a learned task or skill in a new context.

References

General References

Gabbard, C. P. 2008. *Lifelong Motor Development*, 5th ed. San Francisco: Pearson Benjamin Cummings.

Kandel, E. R., J. H. Schwartz, and T. M. Jessell (eds). 1995. *Essentials of Neural Science and Behavior*. New York: McGraw-Hill.

Schmidt, R. A. and T. D. Lee. 2005. *Motor Control and Learning. A Behavioral Approach*, 4th ed. Champaign, IL: Human Kinetics.

Schmidt, R. A., and C. W. Wrisberg. 2000. *Motor Learning and Performance. A Problem-based Approach*, 2nd ed. Champaign, IL: Human Kinetics.

Shea, C. H., and D. L. Wright. 1997. *An Introduction to Human Movement. The Sciences of Physical Education*. Needham Heights, MA: Allyn and Bacon.

Zelaznik, H. N. (ed). 1996. Advances in Motor Learning and Control. Champaign, IL: Human Kinetics.

References to Specific Studies

Bronfenbrenner, U. 1986. "Ecology of the Family as a Context for Human Development: Research Perspectives." *Devel. Psychol.* 22:723–42.

Dietz, V. 2003. "Spinal Cord Pattern Generators for Locomotion." *Clin. Neurophysiol.* 114: 1379–1389.

Gesell, A. 1932. "The Developmental Morphology of Infant Behavior Pattern." *Proc. Nat. Acad. Sci.* 18:139–43.

Gibson, E. J., and A. S. Walker. 1984. "Development of Knowledge of Visual-tactual Affordances of Substances." *Child Devel.* 55:453–60.

Kasch, F. W., J. L. Boyer, P. K. Schmidt, R. H. Wells, J. P. Wallace, L. S. Verity, H. Guy, and D. Schneider. 1999. "Ageing of the Cardiovascular System During 33 Years of Aerobic Exercise." *Age and Ageing* 28:531–35.

Nandi, D., T. Z. Aziz, X. Liu, and J. F. Stein. 2002. "Brainstem Motor Loops in the Control of Movement." *Mov. Disord.* 17 (Suppl 3): S22-S27.

Chapter 6

CLINICAL EXERCISE PHYSIOLOGY

The field of clinical exercise physiology is often considered both an art and a science because we use our knowledge of the scientific bases of how a body responds to exercise and combine it with the less quantitative aspects of how we deal with an individual in real life settings. This individual may have different limitations than another, different health issues and different goals from exercise, and all of these considerations have to be taken into account when testing a person or setting up an exercise program for her. Therefore, we consider clinical exercise physiology to be both an art and a science.

A major source of employment for a clinical exercise physiologist (CEP) is in a cardiorespiratory rehabilitation setting. These may be associated with hospitals, or may be free-standing clinics with a physician attending. CEPs employed in these settings often perform exercise tests and give what are referred to as exercise prescriptions, or plans for exercising to improve health and fitness. CEPs may also work with healthy people who are at risk, such as firefighters or police officers who have stressful positions and are often subject to awkward schedules that may limit their ability to eat a healthy diet or exercise regularly. A major characteristic, though is that they try to work with clients as individuals. This allows them to practice both the art and science of clinical exercise physiology.

An ever larger number of CEPs achieve training and certification through national organizations. The major organization for exercise physiologists is the American College of Sports Medicine (ACSM). The ACSM has two certifications for CEPs. The ACSM Certified Clinical Exercise Specialist[SM], works with clients who may have cardiovascular, pulmonary or metabolic disease or other conditions that limit exercise capacity or increase the risk of exercise. The ACSM Registered Clinical Exercise Physiologist® assists clients being treated by a physician for cardiovascular, pulmonary, metabolic, orthopedic, neuromuscular or immunological disease (ACSM, 2010). The American Society of Exercise Physiologists also provides a certification, the Exercise Physiologist Certified, which is similar in many ways to the clinical exercise specialist. Increasingly, students who desire positions as CEPs will be expected to have one of these certifications or to be working on obtaining it to find a job.

Exercise Testing

A key part of the CEP's job is to perform exercise testing on clients who may be healthy or at risk for cardiovascular, pulmonary or metabolic disease. Exercise tests are performed for three main purposes, functional, diagnostic, and prognostic. These purposes may overlap greatly, as we will see. A functional test is conducted for the purpose of finding the level of fitness of the client. This may take place in a clinical setting, but may also be performed in a school, fitness club, or laboratory. The functional aspect of testing is very common and is performed on a wide range of people from sedentary to highly fit athletes. A diagnostic test can be similar to a functional test, but its main purpose is to find out if there is underlying disease of the client, usually as seen on an electrocardiograph, or ECG. Tests of this nature are usually conducted in a clinical setting, but may be performed in a laboratory setting under the supervision of a physician. The purposes of prognostic testing are to both evaluate progress following the initiation of an exercise program, and to determine the likelihood of a positive (or negative) outcome of an exercise test. There are scales used that estimate the incidence of mortality based on exercise test results. This would be an example of a prognostic test.

Screening for Exercise Testing

Before performing an exercise test it is imperative that screening of the client be undertaken. While the risk of exercise among the apparently healthy population is very low, there is still some risk to exercise for some people, and people who appear to be healthy sometimes have underlying disease. The risk of death and of a myocardial infarction (heart attack) during or briefly following a maximal exercise test is approximately 1 in 10,000 and 4 in 10,000 tests, respectively. Since there are risks to exercise, the goal of the prescreening is to weigh the indications against the contraindications for exercise. Indications are why we do exercise, while contraindications are reasons that we may not want the person to do exercise. The basic goals of pre-screening are as follows:

- To make sure it is safe for an individual to be tested and start an exercise program.
- To determine what type of exercise test is appropriate—maximal vs. submaximal, cycle vs. treadmill, etc.
- To assess what, if any, medical supervision is necessary for the person and for the type of exercise test.

One of the simplest pre-screening tests is the Physical Activity Readiness Questionnaire (PAR-Q). The PAR-Q (Figure 6–1) asks several questions about health and conditions that may be related to diseases, primarily cardiovascular diseases. If all questions are answered "no" then the subject is usually allowed to be tested or to begin an exercise program.

Physical Activity Readiness
Questionnaire - PAR-Q
(revised 2002)

PAR-Q & YOU

(A Questionnaire for People Aged 15 to 69)

Regular physical activity is fun and healthy, and increasingly more people are starting to become more active every day. Being more active is very safe for most people. However, some people should check with their doctor before they start becoming much more physically active.

If you are planning to become much more physically active than you are now, start by answering the seven questions in the box below. If you are between the ages of 15 and 69, the PAR-Q will tell you if you should check with your doctor before you start. If you are over 69 years of age, and you are not used to being very active, check with your doctor.

Common sense is your best guide when you answer these questions. Please read the questions carefully and answer each one honestly: check YES or NO.

YES	NO		
☐	☐	1.	Has your doctor ever said that you have a heart condition <u>and</u> that you should only do physical activity recommended by a doctor?
☐	☐	2.	Do you feel pain in your chest when you do physical activity?
☐	☐	3.	In the past month, have you had chest pain when you were not doing physical activity?
☐	☐	4.	Do you lose your balance because of dizziness or do you ever lose consciousness?
☐	☐	5.	Do you have a bone or joint problem (for example, back, knee or hip) that could be made worse by a change in your physical activity?
☐	☐	6.	Is your doctor currently prescribing drugs (for example, water pills) for your blood pressure or heart condition?
☐	☐	7.	Do you know of <u>any other reason</u> why you should not do physical activity?

If

you

answered

YES to one or more questions

Talk with your doctor by phone or in person BEFORE you start becoming much more physically active or BEFORE you have a fitness appraisal. Tell your doctor about the PAR-Q and which questions you answered YES.

- You may be able to do any activity you want — as long as you start slowly and build up gradually. Or, you may need to restrict your activities to those which are safe for you. Talk with your doctor about the kinds of activities you wish to participate in and follow his/her advice.
- Find out which community programs are safe and helpful for you.

NO to all questions

If you answered NO honestly to <u>all</u> PAR-Q questions, you can be reasonably sure that you can:
- start becoming much more physically active — begin slowly and build up gradually. This is the safest and easiest way to go.
- take part in a fitness appraisal — this is an excellent way to determine your basic fitness so that you can plan the best way for you to live actively. It is also highly recommended that you have your blood pressure evaluated. If your reading is over 144/94, talk with your doctor before you start becoming much more physically active.

DELAY BECOMING MUCH MORE ACTIVE:
- if you are not feeling well because of a temporary illness such as a cold or a fever — wait until you feel better; or
- if you are or may be pregnant — talk to your doctor before you start becoming more active.

PLEASE NOTE: If your health changes so that you then answer YES to any of the above questions, tell your fitness or health professional. Ask whether you should change your physical activity plan.

<u>Informed Use of the PAR-Q</u>: The Canadian Society for Exercise Physiology, Health Canada, and their agents assume no liability for persons who undertake physical activity, and if in doubt after completing this questionnaire, consult your doctor prior to physical activity.

No changes permitted. You are encouraged to photocopy the PAR-Q but only if you use the entire form.

NOTE: If the PAR-Q is being given to a person before he or she participates in a physical activity program or a fitness appraisal, this section may be used for legal or administrative purposes.

"I have read, understood and completed this questionnaire. Any questions I had were answered to my full satisfaction."

NAME _____

SIGNATURE _____ DATE _____

SIGNATURE OF PARENT _____ WITNESS _____
or GUARDIAN (for participants under the age of majority)

Note: This physical activity clearance is valid for a maximum of 12 months from the date it is completed and becomes invalid if your condition changes so that you would answer YES to any of the seven questions.

CSEP | SCPE   © Canadian Society for Exercise Physiology www.csep.ca/forms

FIGURE 6-1. The Physical Activity Readiness Questionnaire.

Source: *Canadian Physical Activity, Fitness & Lifestyle Approach: CSEP-Health & Fitness Program's Appraisal and Counselling Strategy*, 3rd edition, © 2003. Reprinted with permission from the Canadian Society for Exercise Physiology. Source: Physical Activity Readiness Questionnaire (PAR-Q) © 2002. Used with permission from the Canadian Society for Exercise Physiology www.csep.ca.

Activity 6-1.   Take the PAR-Q. How do you rate as far as your ability to start an exercise program? What do each of the questions help the person to understand about his/her ability to begin an exercise program?

In addition to the PAR-Q, many subjects will be asked to fill out a health/medical history questionnaire. This questionnaire can be relatively simple or can consist of many questions and numerous pages. Typically these questionnaires ask about previous diagnosed diseases and hospitalizations, and drugs taken, both prescription and over-the-counter. They will also often ask about family disease history and history of physical activity. This type of questionnaire helps the CEP determine whether further evaluation may be needed by a physician, or may help the physician evaluate results of exercise and other tests that may be given to the client.

In some clients, a physical examination may be required prior to initiating an exercise program or starting a test. This may be expected when the patient is over 45 years for males or 55 for females, if the client has risk factors for cardiovascular or other disease (or a diagnosed disease), or at the discretion of the physician. The physical exam will generally include auscultation (listening to heart and lung sounds), blood pressure and pulse rate, and may include pulmonary function and a resting ECG. Depending on the person, the physical exam may include more comprehensive measures of heart, vessel and lung function, as well as the health of the bones, joints and muscles.

Informed consent

Once it has been determined that a client can be tested, informed consent must be obtained. Informed consent is the process by which we tell the patient what the risks and benefits of the exercise are likely to be. This also tells the client how we will be using the data we collect if we are going to use the data for anything other than to give the patient information. Informed consent must be obtained from the client before any tests are done, usually even before the pre-screening is done. This helps protect the client from possible damaging tests and helps protect the clinician from legal issues.

Types of Testing

Following pre-screening, if an exercise test is warranted, it must be decided what type of test is to be used. Some laboratories and clinics do not vary the testing very much between subjects, while others may offer a wide variety of tests. Most exercise tests are referred to as graded exercise tests (GXTs). It is called this because the test consists of a series of loads or stages through which the subject works. Each load is more difficult than the previous one. Typically the stages are three minutes in length, but can vary from one minute to four to five minutes. The first step in determining the type of test is usually deciding whether to perform a submaximal or maximal test. Submaximal tests generally have lower mortality and morbidity, but may not be as effective at diagnosing a cardiac problem that only shows up on an ECG at a relatively high work load. People with diagnosed diseases are often tested using submaximal protocols, but this is not universal.

In addition to the type of test, we want to decide which mode of testing to use, or what type of exercise. In the Unites States, treadmill walking and running protocols are the most often used. This is because most Americans are more familiar with foot locomotion than any other form of aerobic exercise. The use of a treadmill, though, can become somewhat of a problem for people with orthopedic impediments to the hips, knees and ankles. These subjects may not be able to exert themselves on a treadmill to the intensity required to elicit a maximal effort without pain. Those with balance problems such as some elderly patients or those with impaired neuromuscular control may also not be able to perform a treadmill test. In these patients, the use of a cycle ergometer is often called for. Modes of exercise testing should also be tailored to the individual's preference and training background. For example, bicycle racers will usually yield better results on a cycle ergometer than on a treadmill. There are also ergometers built for rowing and other sports that may be useful for functional testing of athletes in those activities (Figure 6–2).

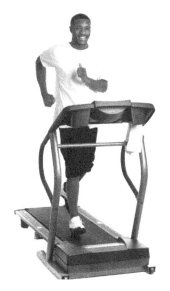
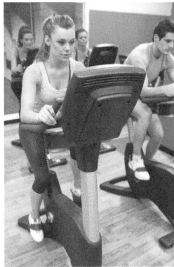
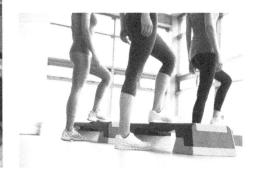

FIGURE 6–2. Examples of different ergonomic testing devices.

© Flashon Studio, 2013. Used under license from Shutterstock, Inc. © wavebreakmedia, 2013. Used under license from Shutterstock, Inc.

Protocols used for exercise testing

One of the most common treadmill testing protocols is the Bruce protocol. This protocol is designed to elicit a maximal effort on the part of the subjects in eight to twelve minutes. The stages are set up so that the test starts at about 4.5 METS. There is approximately a three MET increase in load per stage. One MET, or METabolic equivalent is equivalent to resting metabolic rate, so a person with a 10 MET maximum has a maximal capacity that is ten times resting. With the average sedentary adult having a maximal capacity of ten METs, this elicits a maximal effort in nine minutes. One drawback to this test is that it requires the subject to walk/run at a pace that is too fast for comfortable walking and too slow for comfortable jogging through about two stages, and many do not prefer this. However, there is a great deal of data on the Bruce protocol, it is appropriate for testing one of the widest range of fitness levels of subjects, and it remains one of the most widely used treadmill tests. A second protocol, the Naughton protocol, starts at 2 METs and increases the load at only approximately 1 MET per stage, so is appropriate if you have unfit or diseased clients and still desire that they complete eight to twelve minutes of a test. Another protocol, the Balke-Ware protocol, starts at about 3.5 METs, but increases the load at an even smaller 0.5 METs per stage, making it better for people who are very unfit or have more advanced disease, but can still be tested. Tests such as the Naughton and Balke protocols would not be appropriate for fit subjects because they might complete as much as 20 minutes on the treadmill, which is well outside the desired eight to twelve minutes. Many labs use only one protocol for testing because the range of subjects that they test is relatively small and most complete the desired time on the test. Others change the test protocol based on what is expected of the subject. Figure 6–3 shows the increase in load over time with the three protocols described above.

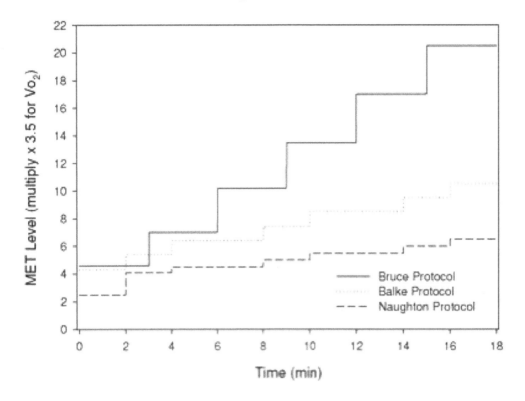

FIGURE 6–3. Bruce, Balke and Naughton protocols used in treadmill testing.

Measurements and interpretations from a GXT

Many measurements are made during a GXT that help us determine both the fitness and the health status of the patient. These measurements range from very simple to complex and expensive. One of the most common is to either measure or estimate maximal oxygen uptake (Vo_2max). Vo_2max is one of the best estimates of aerobic capacity, which is an indicator of the health and fitness of the cardiovascular, respiratory and muscle systems. Ideally, oxygen uptake is measured using a system that measures the ventilation and the amount of O_2 and CO_2 in the inspired and expired air. From these, the Vo_2 is calculated and the highest Vo_2 is taken as the Vo_2max. Vo_2 is measured in L/min or ml/min, also called the absolute Vo_2, and is converted to ml/kg/min by dividing by body weight and converting L/min to ml/min. This is the relative Vo_2 because the Vo_2 is *relative* to body weight, and this gives us a good idea of the fitness of the individual. To measure Vo_2 is complicated, subject to potential error, and is expensive, so we will sometimes estimate the Vo_2 for the stage of the exercise or use the duration of the exercise to predict Vo_2max based on these. This is usually a good method because the stages of the protocols are well known and the amount of oxygen a person should use at each stage is nearly the same for almost all of us. The potential for error is greater using this method, but the test is much less expensive and the error is seldom more than about 10%, which may be acceptable for clinical measures. What do we expect to see regarding Vo_2max in a client? Typically Vo_2 will increase with each stage until the client has achieved a maximal exertion, then it will not increase any further (Figure 6–4). Table 6–1 shows values for men and women of various fitness levels. These are only examples, but will give you an idea of the range for an individual. Vo_2max will be lower in diseased people and it declines with age after about 30 years. It is also typically about 10% lower in women than men of similar fitness categories.

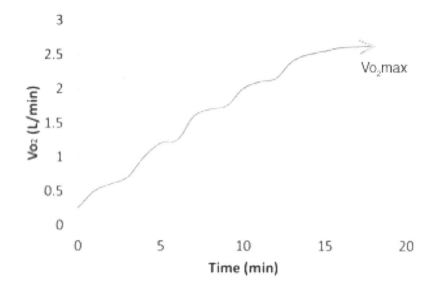

FIGURE 6–4. Response of Vo_2 to workloads up to Vo_2max.

TABLE 6–1. Typical values seen for Vo_2max among different populations. Units are ml/kg/min.

Fitness Category	Men	Women
Aged or with disease	<25	<20
Sedentary	30–40	25–35
Fit	45–55	40–50
Elite	>70	>65

We also measure heart rate and blood pressure during a GXT. Similar to the changes in Vo_2, we expect heart rate to increase with each stage until maximal exertion. We can estimate maximal heart rate using the formula:

$$\text{Max HR} = 220 - \text{age (yrs)}$$

There is a great potential for error using this formula since it is based on a population, but it gives one a place to start. If at the end of a test, the person is within 10 beats/min of the estimated max HR, then we can usually assume that this was a test that caused the subject to make a maximal effort. Heart rate can be measured using palpation at the wrist, or using a heart rate monitor or electrocardiograph (ECG) machine. Heart rate may be measured continuously through the test or at the end of each stage.

Blood pressure is measured during a GXT to give an indication of both heart and blood vessel function. A typical response of blood pressure during exercise is for systolic to increase in proportion to the exercise intensity, but for diastolic to stay approximately the same. It may also decrease slightly in some people. Systolic pressure increases with the increased pumping of the heart,
but diastolic doesn't increase much because the vessels in the body, particularly in the muscles,
dilate during exercise to enable them to withstand the increased amount of blood flowing through
them. An increase in systolic pressure to over 250 mmHg, or a decrease in systolic pressure with
increased work may be a reason to stop a test. A graph of a typical blood pressure and heart rate
response to exercise is shown in Figure 6–5.

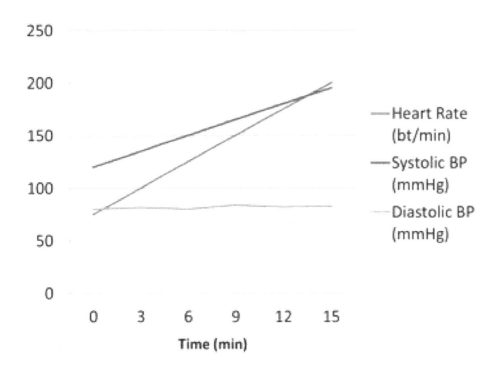

FIGURE 6-5. Changes in heart rate, systolic and diastolic pressure during an incremental exercise test.

An electrocardiogram (ECG or EKG) is often measured during a diagnostic or prognostic test
to help determine whether the heart depolarizes normally as its work increases. An ECG uses positive and negative electrodes to record the electrical activity of the heart. Electrodes are placed on the
subject so that there are 12 leads or combinations of positive and negative electrodes. These "look"
at the heart from different directions and allow the physician or ECG technician to evaluate the

activity while the test is ongoing. There are characteristic changes in the ECG that are associated with some relatively common problems, like ischemia, or insufficient blood flow to the coronary arteries serving the heart itself. These are very important, since blockage of one or more of these arteries may cause a myocardial infarction, or heart attack. In a test, the ECG is monitored while the subject is supine at rest, standing at rest, during each exercise stage, and for six to ten minutes following the test. Figure 6–6 shows examples of two typical ECGs, one normal and one with signs of ischemia.

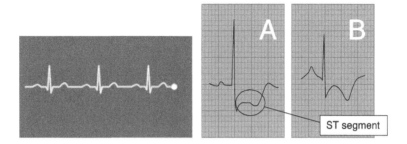

FIGURE 6-6. Normal and abnormal ECG examples. Note the segment immediately following the QRS complex is below the baseline in the example on the right. This is a sign of ischemia.

© Inge Sherpers, 2013. Used under license from Shutterstock, Inc. © Kendall Hunt Publishing

There are also a number of readings taken during many GXTs that are perceptual in nature. That is, they ask the patient to rate his level of pain, exertion, or difficulty in exercise. The most common of these is the rating of perceived exertion (RPE), sometimes called the Borg scale after its developer. This scale ranges from 6–20 or 0–10 (6–20 is more common) and simply asks the client to list how hard she feels the exercise is at that moment. The scale is useful in getting the patient to think about how hard an exercise bout is and how hard the exercise should be. For example, the CEP may ask the subject to exercise for 20 minutes at a heart rate of 130–150. Monitoring heart rate is often difficult for clients, but with a little practice, it is relatively simple to exercise to a certain RPE level. An example of a RPE scale can be seen in Figure 6–7. The RPE scale was designed to reflect heart rate, but remove the 0, so that a heart rate of 140 would yield an RPE of approximately 14. Therefore, in many people an RPE of 13–15 would arise at a heart rate of 130–150, but this is very individual, so the relationship should be established for each client. Similar scales exist for angina or chest pain, and for dyspnea, or breathing difficulty. Both of these are commonly used when testing patients who either have or are suspected of having cardiac or respiratory disease, but are not commonly used for fitness testing or for general diagnostic testing when disease is not likely to be present or limiting.

RPE Scale

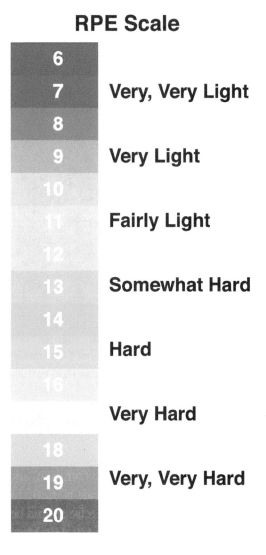

FIGURE 6-7. Example of Borg's RPE scale with word cues.
© Kendall Hunt Publishing

Exercise Prescription

Following the completion of the exercise test and its interpretation, it is common to implement an exercise plan or exercise prescription. An exercise prescription is a plan for exercise specifically designed for an individual based on her exercise test and assessment information. Most of what we will be talking about in this section involves a cardiorespiratory exercise prescription designed to improve aerobic capacity and endurance. One of the keys to the exercise prescription is that it is individualized. While there are guidelines for exercise prescriptions and some general principles that are followed, they are set up for specific people based on their needs and goals. There are three primary goals of an exercise prescription. These are to improve health, increase physical working capacity and to ensure safety.

Exercise has been shown to both reduce the risk of disease and decrease the severity of the disease, particularly cardiovascular and certain metabolic diseases. Recent evidence, for example, has shown that reducing body fat through exercise decreases the need for insulin in type II diabetics (Bacchi, et. al., 2012, Lee, et. al., 2011). Some studies have also suggested that blockage of coronary arteries can be decreased through exercise, thus reducing the likelihood of a heart attack or myocardial infarction (Thijssen, et. al., 2012). Therefore, an exercise prescription is likely to have the effect of reducing the risk of some diseases in healthy and at-risk subjects, and reduce the severity or progression of disease in people who have been diagnosed with many cardiovascular and metabolic diseases.

Exercise definitely increases physical capacity if done properly. Many studies show an increase in Vo_2max and the percent of Vo_2max that a person can maintain for a prolonged period of time. They also show an increase in strength, muscle mass and muscle endurance following training compared to pre-training. This is the basis of a proper training program, whether for a team sport, elite athletes, or clinical patients.

Finally, it is imperative that an exercise prescription be given to a subject while taking into account their specific strengths and weaknesses. We will discuss some specifics later in the chapter, but some of the things to take into account include the initial level of fitness, and the presence/absence/severity of disease. These can be very important in setting initial levels of intensity for different exercises. We also want to take into consideration the subject's specific conditions that may make certain exercises difficult, like arthritis, injuries, or balance issues that may make weight bearing or other exercises potentially dangerous for one client that would be perfectly appropriate for another.

Training Principles

Regardless of how we set up an exercise prescription, there are several principles of training that need to be taken into account. Two of the main principles of training are specificity and overload. The principle of specificity says that we need to exercise certain muscle groups, specific metabolic systems (aerobic/anaerobic) and use actions that we want to train for the system to respond appropriately. For example, marathon runners spend very little, if any, time doing 100m sprints in practice. They need to stress their aerobic system in order for it to experience an improvement. The overload principle says that we need to stress or overload the system in order for it to respond. Basically, if we have little or no difficulty doing ten bench presses with 100 pounds (~45 kg), then doing a bench press workout with 100 pounds or less, unless with increased number of repetitions, will not lead to an improvement. We must overload the system.

Two other training principles are not always included, but are extremely important. These are the principles of regression and of individuality of response. Regression is more commonly known as detraining. If we do not stress the system, it will not only not improve, but may decrease in its ability to perform. We see this in the off-season for many athletes who do not train adequately. Individuality of response is central to the exercise prescription. We know that not all people have the same goals, the same starting point in terms of condition, or the same rate of improvement. Therefore, we have to take these into account when helping someone develop an individualized training program. A person who has the goal of becoming a competitive cyclist will be much more willing to work hard at training than a person with the goal of cycle commuting. Further, a person with disease needs to be monitored very closely in some cases in order to prevent themselves from exercising too hard, too long, or too often and causing a worsening of the disease.

FITT principle

When we design an exercise program we manipulate the frequency, intensity, duration, and mode of the exercise bouts. Increasing any of these variables can lead to improvements in condition through the specificity and overload principles. The FITT principle incorporates these variables. FITT is an acronym for Frequency, Intensity, Time (=duration) and Type (=mode).

Frequency is how often we do exercise. Usually this is the number of times per week, but in some cases it can be the number of times per day, with the assumption that it is done on most or all days of the week. Most researchers agree that frequency needs to be on most or all days of the week, but improvements are seen in some individuals with only three days per week of exercise.

Intensity is how hard we do the exercise. It is typically expressed as the percent of Vo_2max or percent of HRmax at which we work during the exercise. Some use the rating of perceived exertion to evaluate intensity and allow the subject to self-pace. To use heart rate to assign intensity, we usually use a percentage of what is termed heart rate reserve (HRR). HRR is the difference between resting and maximal heart rate, or how much heart rate can increase during exercise. We usually use a percent of HRR to determine exercise intensity because it correlates well with the percent of Vo_2max. At 50% of HRR, the client will be exercising at nearly 50% of Vo_2max. The target heart rate, or heart rate at which we desire to exercise is the percent of HRR determined by the exercise test, plus the resting heart rate. Let's work through an example, given the following known values:

Resting HR = 60 bt/min, Maximal HR = 200 bt/min

The exercise is prescribed at a range of 50%–70% of Vo_2max or 50%–70% HRR

What is the target heart rate?

HRR = 200 bt/min − 60 bt/min = 140 bt/min

50% HRR = 140 bt/min × 0.50 = 70 bt/min
70% HRR = 140 bt/min × 0.70 = 98 bt/min

Target HR = 60 bt/min + 70 bt/min = 130 bt/min as the lower target HR
                    60 bt/min + 98 bt/min = 158 bt/min as the higher target HR

So the exercise target heart rate is between 130 and 158 bt/min

Intensity varies greatly across exercise prescriptions, mainly based on the initial fitness level of the patient. For unfit subjects a starting intensity may be as low as 30% Vo_2max, while for a fit person it can be as high as 75–90% Vo_2max.

Time is how long we exercise. This is usually given in minutes, but can be a distance (e.g., a two mile jog). It can also be the number of repetitions and sets in a resistance training program. Typical exercise prescriptions have durations of 20–60 minutes, with a minimum of 20 minutes generally recommended. For people who are very deconditioned either due to sedentary lifestyle or disease it is sometimes recommended to break the exercise into several periods of as little as five to ten minutes, achieving a total of 20 or more minutes in a day.

Type is the mode of exercise. A great many exercise prescriptions will start with walking or stationary cycling as an initial mode of exercise because this allows ready monitoring of the client, but the exercise prescription for cardiorespiratory fitness can encompass almost any mode of aerobic exercise that provides a sufficient stress on the body. By changing the type, it may also make the exercise more enjoyable for the patient, so that he does not get as bored by doing the same thing for weeks at a time.

Rate of progression

A key to the overload principle described above is understanding about progression during training. Progression refers to how rapidly we increase the volume of training. We can increase the total training volume by increasing any or all of the components of training, intensity, duration and frequency. In general, the ten percent rule is a good starting point. That is, we should not increase the volume of exercise by more than about 10% per week. Volume is the combination of frequency, duration and intensity. That means that if you increase the intensity, you generally should not increase the frequency or duration at the same time. If we go back to the idea of individuality of response as one of the training principles, it is important to note that this 10% rule is variable. If, for example, we set the initial exercise prescription very low out of caution for the patient, we may find that she is better able to tolerate the exercise than we suspected and we can increase intensity and duration in some cases by more than a total of 10%. On the other hand, if the patient has difficulty with the exercise prescribed, it may require not increasing any component of the training regimen for two or more weeks, until the client is able to tolerate the load.

The Basic Exercise Prescription

While there are an almost infinite variety of exercise prescriptions, or even initial exercise prescriptions, if one uses the principles described above, the prescription will usually work. Based on the principles and guidelines, an initial exercise prescription similar to the one described below will be a good starting point.

This exercise prescription is for a 35 year old sedentary male without known heart or other disease. This person has the goal to lose some weight (20–40 pounds) and to get in good enough aerobic shape to complete a 5k run within six months. His initial Vo_2max was estimated to be 30 ml/kg/min and his resting and maximal heart rates were 72 and 182, respectively. The general guidelines for someone this low in terms of fitness are to start with a relatively low intensity, but maintain a higher frequency and duration (if tolerable) to make up for the low intensity and allow for an appropriate target volume of exercise. We also want a low intensity to make sure if there is some disease present that he will not be harmed.

Initial Exercise Prescription

Intensity, 30–40% HRR
Duration 20–30 min per day
Frequency 4–5 days per week

We would be careful about following the 10% rule for at least three to four weeks, while he got accustomed to the exercise routine. Following several weeks at this level we would want to re-evaluate him to make sure the load was not too easy or too difficult, and that he had complied with the program. If he found this too easy, we would increase the intensity and duration, but leave the frequency at this level, still following the 10% rule.

Special Considerations for Exercise Testing and Prescription

It is important to note that the program we have outlined above is for a healthy younger person, who is simply sedentary and deconditioned. There are many other conditions that require an adjustment to the exercise prescription. Most of these adjustments are modifications of intensity or mode of exercise to accommodate a patient's specific medical or other issues that affect exercise.

Diabetes

Diabetes is one of the most common metabolic disorders. It is an impaired ability to take up glucose due to either a deficiency in the ability of the pancreas to produce insulin or the ability of the cells to react to insulin that is produced, or both. Type 1 diabetes, often called childhood diabetes, mostly begins at a young age, but can occur at any time. It is characterized by a lack of ability to produce insulin, so glucose builds up in the blood. It is treated with insulin as well as being managed with appropriate dietary manipulations. Type 2 diabetes, often called adult onset diabetes and mostly seen in obese inactive people is becoming increasingly common in young people. It is characterized by insulin resistance at the cells, but can also include decreased insulin production. It is often treated by diet modifications and decrease in body weight, but in some people requires insulin as well. Both types of diabetes appear to be increasing in the population within the United States, but type 2 diabetes is much more common and increasing along with the increase in the obesity incidence. Some good news, though, is that type 2 diabetes may actually be treated with exercise and weight loss and some diabetics can see the disease disappear through these interventions.

A person with uncontrolled diabetes may be harmed by exercise. Thus uncontrolled diabetes is referred to as a relative contraindication. Therefore careful screening by a physician is required prior to initiating an exercise program. This screening should include a GXT, since cardiovascular disease is more likely to be present in diabetic subjects than in the population as a whole. Once cleared to do exercise, the exercise prescription usually follows similar guidelines to the healthy population. Special consideration needs to be given to the abnormal glucose responses of diabetics, so during the initial stage of the program, the patient is usually monitored for signs and symptoms of exercise intolerance and for blood glucose levels. Type 2 diabetics are often obese, so carefully monitoring intensity may be increasingly important in this group, and initial exercise prescriptions may stress more the frequency and duration rather than the intensity to decrease the likelihood of injury. Obese subjects may also be encouraged to do less weight bearing activities, things like stationary cycling and water activities.

Cardiovascular diseases

Hypertension is the most prevalent cardiovascular disease in the western world. Hypertension is defined as a systolic blood pressure over 140 mmHg or a diastolic pressure over 90 mmHg. The vast majority of hypertension is termed essential, which means no specific cause. Secondary hypertension is usually a result of dysfunction of the kidneys or of the endocrine (hormone) system. Treatment of essential hypertension is accomplished through drug interventions, dietary manipulation (lower sodium intake in some people, for example), weight loss and exercise. Therefore, exercise is a major factor in the modification of the disease, and may actually lower blood pressure. The exercise prescription is very similar to those in otherwise healthy people, that is three to seven days/week at an intensity of 40%–70% HRR with a duration of about 30+ minutes. Some special considerations that may apply to some hypertensive patients include those you would apply if the person was obese, as above. Also, if the person is severely hypertensive, it is often recommended to have them on medication that has lowered and stabilized the blood pressure prior to initiating the exercise prescription.

Heart failure is the inability of the heart to pump adequate amounts of blood to the system. This can be due to a disease that has rendered the heart muscle incapable of contracting. It can also be a result of prolonged hypertension that has weakened the heart. With the aging of the population, heart failure has increased greatly, and is a leading cause of hospitalization for people 65 and older. The primary early symptom is intolerance for exercise that is unexpected along with fatigue and breathlessness. Peripheral edema or swelling may also occur. Treatment is often with medications that either decrease peripheral resistance, making it easier for the heart to pump, or drugs that increase the force of the heartbeat. Heart transplants are also effective treatments for heart failure, but the lack of availability of donor hearts decreases the likelihood of getting this type of treatment. Exercise tolerance is decreased dramatically in heart failure, so exercise prescriptions may be difficult. Still, many clinical trials have been performed to determine the best prescriptions for these patients. Cardiovascular conditioning is a primary objective in heart failure, and cycle ergometry or walking are often used as the modes of exercise. These provide sufficient intensity and the ability to grade the intensity to the subject, but also help in acts of daily living. It is generally suggested that the patient be stable on her medications prior to initiating an exercise program.

Respiratory diseases

Chronic obstructive pulmonary disease (COPD) consists of chronic bronchitis and emphysema. These diseases cause a narrowing or destruction of the airways, making it difficult to breathe, particularly to exhale (Figure 6–8). Most cases are due to cigarette smoking, with less than 1% having emphysema due to a genetic defect. Passive smoke exposure, air pollution and occupational exposures also contribute to the disease in some people. Exercise is difficult in people with COPD, and the inability to perform exercise that was once routine without undue breathlessness is one of the symptoms that often brings COPD patients in to the physician and leads to a diagnosis. COPD is related to pack-years (one pack year = smoking an average of one pack of cigarettes per day for one year) of smoking, so is often not seen until later in life. For this reason, many patients delay seeking treatment since they blame the decrease in their ability to exercise simply on the aging process until the disease has progressed sufficiently to limit exertion by itself. Numerous drugs are given to decrease inflammation in the airways and to dilate them, which improve exercise capacities, but the disease does not have any known cure and progresses to the point of mortality. Exercise prescription depends on the severity of the disease. An exercise prescription for COPD generally consists of exercises to tolerance along with specific exercises for the respiratory muscles to help strengthen them. Supplemental oxygen is often given during exercise, even if it is not required for daily activities, in order to make the exertion more comfortable.

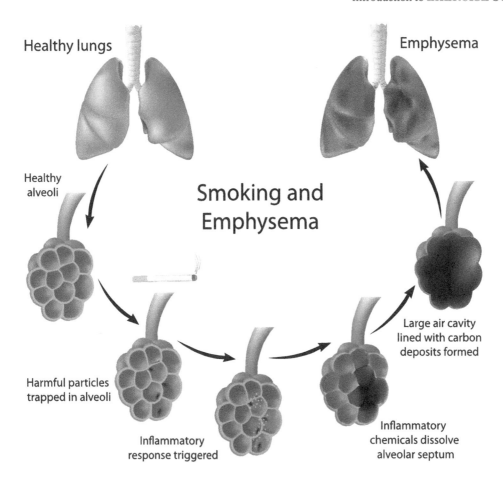

FIGURE 6-8. Progression of disease in emphysema.
© Alila Medical Images, 2013. Used under license from Shutterstock, Inc.

Asthma is a narrowing of the airways, but is due to hyperactivity of the smooth muscle in the airways. While the disease may be long term, it is characterized by acute bouts of breathing difficulty, sometimes to the extent that death results if not adequately treated (Figure 6–9). Asthma attacks can be brought about by allergens such as dust or foods, by exercise, by stress or other factors. Treatment is generally by drugs, either acute or long-term, and by manipulation of the factors that precipitate attacks, such as avoiding exposure to substances to which the person is allergic, or timing exercise to avoid conditions such as cold or air pollution. Exercise prescriptions for asthma vary tremendously based on the severity of the disease and what brings on the attacks. It is important, though, to monitor symptoms of breathlessness during exercise because many people with asthma also exhibit asthma symptoms during exercise. Therefore it is often suggested that asthmatic subjects carry their acute medications with them. Early in an exercise program it is often suggested to have continuous monitoring by a professional until the patient knows what the onset of symptoms feels like and can take action on her own.

Pathology of Asthma

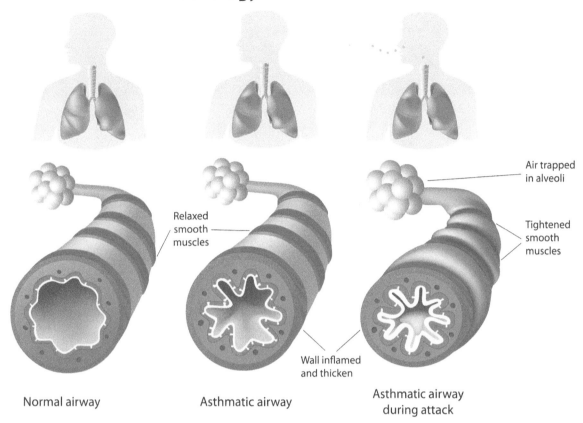

FIGURE 6–9. Airways of a healthy person, an asthmatic and an asthmatic during an attack.
© Alila Medical Images, 2013. Used under license from Shutterstock, Inc.

Arthritis

Arthritis is a degenerative disease of the joints and affects comfort and range of movement, thus affecting exercise capacity (Figure 6–10). There are two types of arthritis, osteoarthritis and rheumatoid arthritis. **Osteoarthritis** is the more common of the two types and is often associated with age and previous injury or overuse of a joint. **Rheumatoid arthritis** is usually considered an autoimmune disease, in which the body attacks itself, resulting in joint damage and destruction. Treatments include non-steroidal anti-inflammatory drugs (NSAIDs) such as aspirin, ibuprofen and acetaminophen and progress to stronger anti-inflammatory drugs such as corticosteroids. For rheumatoid arthritis, drugs that suppress the immune system are also often prescribed. Exercise prescriptions have to take into account the severity of the disease and the specific joints affected, so as not to aggravate the symptoms. Therefore a person will often be prescribed non-weight bearing exercises if the damage is to the lower limbs. It is important that the inflammation be managed prior to initiating the exercise program to avoid accelerating the progress of the disease. This appears to be particularly true in rheumatoid arthritis. Flexibility exercises are often prescribed to increase the range of motion in addition to exercises to improve fitness.

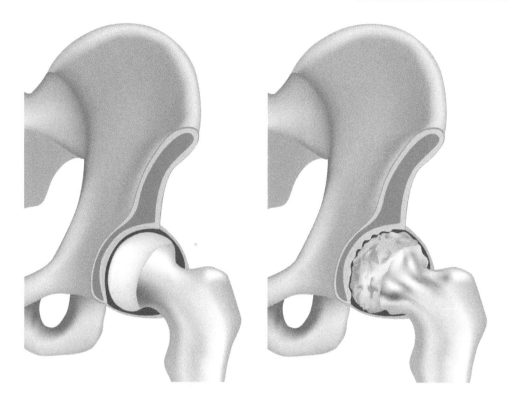

Healthy hip joint   Osteoarthritis

FIGURE 6-10. Arthritic joint shows damage to the joint caused by overuse.
© Alila Medical Images, 2013. Used under license from Shutterstock, Inc.

Conclusions

The primary objectives of exercise testing are to assess the level of fitness, to diagnose disease if present and to make a prediction about the outcome (prognosis) of the person based on the disease and the exercise treatment. Exercise tests are performed to maximize the ability to achieve these objectives while minimizing the risk of injury or death to the subject. There are numerous types of tests that can be performed based on the health and fitness level of the subject and his/her specific interests and preferences in exercise.

An exercise prescription is a personalized exercise program based on the results of screenings and the exercise tests performed. The goals of an exercise prescription are to improve health, to improve exercise capacity and to ensure the safety of the client, both during and following the exercise. While there are many commonalities between exercise prescriptions, there are differences as well, based on the specific fitness of the individual as well as diseases that may be present, and all these affect how we assign exercise to a patient.

Glossary

Arthritis—disease of the joints that results in inflammation and degradation of the joint.

Asthma—disease of the airways in which airways narrow because of hyperactivity of the smooth muscle of the airways.

Chronic obstructive pulmonary disease—narrowing of the airways. Specifically this refers to chronic bronchitis and emphysema. Also called COPD.

Contraindication—a reason not to perform an activity, in this case a reason not to do an exercise test or prescribe exercise.

Diabetes—impaired ability to take up glucose, either due to a deficiency in insulin production or a decreased ability of the cells to react to insulin.

Diagnostic exercise test—test performed to determine presence or absence of disease.

Electrocardiogram—electrical recording of activity of the heart.

Exercise Prescription—a plan for exercise designed for an individual based on a previous exercise test and assessment.

FITT principle—frequency, intensity, time and type of exercise.

Functional exercise test—test performed to assess fitness level.

Graded exercise test—an exercise test performed in increasing stages or levels of exercise intensity.

Heart failure—inability of the heart to pump adequate amounts of blood to the body.

Hypertension—elevated resting blood pressure, usually considered as greater than 140/90.

Indication—a reason to perform an activity, in this case a reason one should perform an exercise test or begin an exercise program.

Informed consent—means by which we describe the process and likely outcomes of a procedure to a patient.

Maximal oxygen uptake—highest ability to take in and use oxygen in the body. This is one of the best indicators of aerobic fitness.

Metabolic equivalent—multiple of resting metabolic rate. It is used to estimate exercise intensity. Also called a MET.

Overload—a principle of training that states one must stress the system to increase its ability.

Oxygen uptake—the amount of oxygen taken up and used by the body during an activity.

Physical activity readiness questionnaire—a baseline level screening test performed prior to an exercise test or program. Also called PAR-Q.

Prognostic exercise test—test performed to assess the likelihood of mortality or morbidity, or to evaluate the progress of training during an exercise prescription.

Rating of perceived exertion—assessment of exercise intensity that relies on the individual's feeling of the exercise at that time. Also termed RPE.

Regression—a principle of training that states if training is stopped or decreased, the body responds by decreasing its ability, also referred to as detraining.

Specificity—a principle of training that states the body responds to the specific stress put on it, for example leg vs. arm exercise or spring vs. endurance exercise.

References

General References

American College of Sports Medicine. 2010. *ACSM's Guidelines for Exercise Testing and Prescription*, 8th ed. Philadelphia: Wolters Kluwer Health.

American College of Sports Medicine. 2010. *ACSM's Resource Manual for Guidelines for Exercise Testing and Prescription,* 6th ed. Philadelphia: Wolters Kluwer Health.

Crouse, S. F. and J. R. Coast. 2011. *Clinical Exercise Physiology Laboratory Manual*, 2nd ed. Dubuque, IA: Kendall Hunt.

Ehrman, J. K., P. M. Gordon, P. S. Visich, and S. J. Keteyian. 2003. *Clinical Exercise Physiology.* Champaign, IL: Human Kinetics.

Heyward, V. J. 2002. *Advanced Fitness Assessment and Exercise Prescription*, 4th ed. Champaign, IL: Human Kinetics.

References to Specific Studies

Bacchi, E, C. Negri, M. E. Zanolin, C. Milanese, N. Faccioli, M. Trombetta, G. Zoppini, et. al., 2012. "Metabolic Effects of Aerobic Training and Resistance Training in Type 2 Diabetic Subjects: A Randomized Controlled Trial (the RAED2 study)." *Diabetes Care* 35:676–82.

Lee, S., Y. Park and C. Zhang. 2011. "Exercise Training Prevents Coronary Endothelial Dysfunction in Type 2 Diabetic Mice." *Am. J. Biomed. Sci.* 3:241–52.

Thijssen, D. H. J., N. T. Cable and D. J. Green. 2012. "Impact of Exercise Training on Arterial Wall Thickness in Humans." *Clin. Sci.* 122:311–22.

Chapter 7
HEALTH, FITNESS, AND WELLNESS

The areas of health and fitness are viewed by many as a branch of exercise physiology, which we discussed in another chapter. There is no question that health, fitness, and wellness practitioners need a background in physiology in order to understand their field. To understand why fitness lowers cardiovascular death risk, it is important to know the cardiovascular responses to exercise, as well as the metabolism of fats and cholesterol. It is more, though, than exercise physiology. An expert in health and wellness also needs to have an understanding of kinesiology to fully comprehend muscle fitness, an understanding of epidemiology to follow studies performed and the conclusions that are drawn from them, and an understanding of exercise psychology to help motivate others to exercise.

Compared to fields such as exercise physiology and kinesiology, the profession of health and fitness in exercise is relatively new and its real importance is still being discovered. With the tremendous increases in obesity and the growth of the older population, though, it is an area that is increasing in its need. The explosive growth in health and fitness has led to many positive innovations such as corporate fitness. Parks and recreation services within cities now include fitness centers, nutrition advice, and other amenities and services rather than simply softball fields and picnic areas. Fitness facilities are now more than simply gyms designed for bodybuilders, and are usually staffed with exercise professionals who are certified by organizations such as the American College of Sports Medicine (ACSM) or the American Council on Exercise (ACE). Many of these professionals also have some background in nutrition, allowing them to help with exercise programs and dietary goals at the same time.

The explosion in the field has led to some problems, though. We see many infomercials for questionable products to improve fitness, lower body fat, and generally improve health. It is important to be able to distinguish between fitness professionals who are genuinely knowledgeable and interested in the health of their clients and entrepreneurs who are interested in your wallet, and use fitness as a hook to sell anything from weight loss pills to exercise videos and fancy diets.

Health, Fitness, and Wellness Defined

The terms health, fitness, and wellness all have meanings that separate them, but all are highly related and often used interchangeably. In its strictest definition, health is simply the absence of disease. More globally it is used in terms of physical, mental, and social health. That is, a healthy person is absent of disease, both physical and mental, and is "well adjusted" socially. This usually involves having a family and friends who are both supported and supportive, and a level of stress that is not so high that it interferes with the ability of a person to work well in one's surroundings. Fitness generally relates more to physical health. A person who is able to carry out activities required of him is said to be fit. We often extend this to measures of physical ability, so that a person who is stronger, or has a higher Vo$_2$max, is said to be more fit than one with lower abilities. This makes sense because if the requirement for performing activities increases, the person we have described as being of higher fitness will be better able to perform the new, increased, level of activity. Wellness is a concept that combines health and fitness, as well as the intellectual, spiritual, and environmental aspects of life. It is often viewed as a pie, with each of the pieces contributing to the wellness of the individual, as seen in Figure 7–1. In general, we think of fitness as a physical concept, while wellness encompasses all aspects of life.

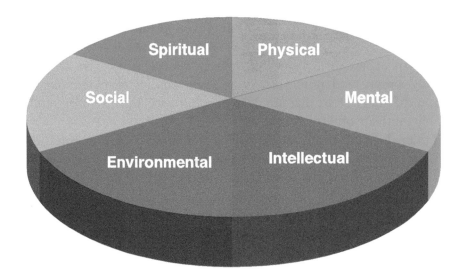

FIGURE 7–1. The different aspects of wellness: physical, mental, social, intellectual, environmental, and spiritual.

Activity 7–1.   List at least four things that contribute to each of the areas of wellness, both in a positive and in a negative way?

Periodically, the U.S. government comes forth with a new set of health goals for the people of the country. These are not mandates, but goals set forth by the most knowledgeable health professionals in the country. You can see that the goals primarily address physical health and decreasing disease, but is there anything in these goals about the mental, social, environmental, intellectual, and spiritual aspects of wellness? Can these be implied in some of the goals? Why might some not have been addressed specifically? Below are the goals of *Healthy People 2020*:

Activity 7–2.   Examine the Healthy People 2020 goals and the background behind them. Are there any of these you think unnecessary? Are there any you would add to it?

Overarching Goals

- Attain high-quality, longer lives free of preventable disease, disability, injury, and premature death.
- Achieve health equity, eliminate disparities, and improve the health of all groups.
- Create social and physical environments that promote good health for all.
- Promote quality of life, healthy development, and healthy behaviors across all life stages.

http://www.healthypeople.gov/2020/about/default.aspx

Quality of Life as a Part of Health, Fitness, and Wellness

Health and fitness are related to both the quantity of life, how long we live, and to the quality of life or how healthy and able to carry on our normal activities we are while we are alive. This is becoming an increasing concern in society. The reason for this concern is not only a compassionate one, in that we prefer to live a long and healthy life and have those around us do so as well. It is also an economic one. Almost daily on the news or other media, the issue of the aging of the population is mentioned. With the aging of the "baby boomers," those born between 1946 and 1964, one of the largest generations in American history is leaving the workforce and entering the age when there is an increased need for health care. If we can keep the population healthy and fit, we reduce the need for some of the expensive medical care associated with aging, and we also reduce the expenses associated with older people needing assistance in nearly everything they do, even if they are not ill. Many studies have examined the effects of fitness on longevity and most come to similar conclusions. Fitness may increase the life span or it may not, but it certainly is associated with a decreased need for expensive care later in life, and the period before death that the person needs expensive care is decreased, meaning that they are ill for less time prior to death. The population of the United States has done this. Figure 7–2 shows survival rates from 1900–2002 at different ages. Through advances in infant mortality between 1900 and 1950, you can see that the survival rate of all ages has improved in the last century. However, you can also see that the slope of the curve from ages zero to about 60 has decreased as well, with many more people living to age 60 now, than even in 1950. This is mainly due to improvements in prevention of food-borne illnesses and medical care. We see similar, although not as dramatic, curves when comparing fit vs. sedentary individuals. In this section, we will cover three specific areas in which exercise and quality/quantity of life have been evaluated, exercise and cardiovascular disease, exercise and aging, and exercise and cancer.

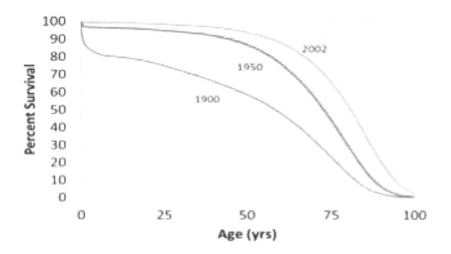

FIGURE 7–2. Survival curves for the US population in 1900, 1950, and 2002. Note that approximately ¾ of the population lived to age 75 in 2002, compared to about 20% in 1900.

(Based on data from the National Vital Statistics Reports, 2004)

Cardiovascular Disease and the Framingham Heart Study

One of the largest and most famous longitudinal studies of lifespan and quality of life is the Framingham Heart Study. Begun in 1948, the study has enrolled three generations of participants (nearly 15,000 people) and continues today under the guidance of the National Institutes of Health. The purpose of the study was to evaluate causes and contributors to the number one killer of Americans, heart disease. They evaluated participants for diet, activity, alcohol consumption, and many other factors, then followed their progress for over 60 years and determined a relationship between these and other factors and the development of heart disease, and death from heart disease and other factors. Among other contributions, the Framingham heart study was one of the first to conclude that exercise could prevent, or at least lessen the onset of coronary disease (Morris, et al., 1973). Other findings that have come out of the Framingham Heart Study include the increased risk of heart disease in obese people (Hubert, et. al, 1983), the effect of cholesterol and blood lipids on the development of heart disease (Castelli, 1988), and the association of diabetes with heart disease (Fox, et. al, 2008; Levitsky, et. al., 2008). The study is now employing research on the genome to evaluate genetic factors in the development of heart disease. You can see from this short description, that studies such as this have spawned a great many ideas about heart disease, exercise, and health that we now take for granted, but were virtually unknown only 40 years ago.

Other studies have found many interesting benefits of even moderate exercise. At the Cooper Clinic in Dallas, Texas, they actually measured fitness levels in thousands of people. From these tests, they divided the subjects into five groups based on fitness. One of the major findings of these studies was that simply doing enough exercise to get **out of the bottom fifth (20%)** decreased all-cause mortality by approximately 50% (Blair, et. al., 1989).

While we discussed diabetes in the Clinical Exercise Physiology chapter, it is important to note that the obesity epidemic in the United States is highly related to the increase in type 2 diabetes. Preventing obesity, through exercise and diet, can almost completely eliminate type 2 diabetes. By decreasing diabetes, we also decrease the risk of heart and vascular diseases that are the leading cause of death in the United States.

Aging and Exercise

Improved fitness is often associated with an increase in the ability to perform exercise and activities of daily living (ADL) for a longer period later in life. Aging, of course, is a natural occurrence, but the debilitation that comes with age is much less so. Take, for example, the records for the marathon. The men's record for 70 years and older is under 2:55 (a whopping pace of 6:40 per mile, Figure 7–3) while that for women is 3:45 (8:40 per mile). How many 20–25 year old people do you suppose can run that fast for 26.2 miles (ref: http://www.arrs.net/SA_Mara. htm)? The reasons that the regression in performance with aging appears to be decreased in fit people are many. As mentioned above, one of the biggest improvements as we age in fit people is in the decrease in heart disease. This is not only one of the major causes of mortality in the United States and other western countries, it is one of the primary causes of disability through strokes, non-fatal heart attacks and other complications. Therefore, decreasing the onset of heart disease should make us better able to perform exercise as well as ADL later in life.

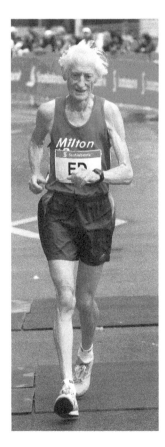

FIGURE 7–3. Ed Whitlock, record holder in the marathon for runners over 70 years.
© Toronto Star via Getty Images.

Another hypothesis as to why people who maintain an exercise program are able to continue physically productive lives longer than those who do not is related to byproducts of aerobic metabolism called reactive oxygen species (ROS, also called free radicals) and the ability to deal with them. ROS are highly reactive chemically, so they can combine with many other substances in the body. ROS are produced during aerobic metabolism and the body has numerous ways of getting rid of them. One theory of aging is that ROS increase in cells and cause damage to those cells and tissues (Muller, et. al., 2007). As the cells replicate, they are thought to pass this damaged DNA to the new cells, and thus the damage appears to accumulate through cell generations, leading to decreased function and decreased life span. With training we may actually produce more ROS due to the increased activity, but we also dramatically increase our production of enzymes that get rid of or scavenge the ROS in the cell. By doing this we may delay the damage to the cell and maintain its function for longer durations during our lives. A similar idea revolves around the inflammation hypothesis (Carter, et. al, 2007), which proposes that as we age we produce more inflammatory agents in the body and these lead to more rapid cell damage and death. Exercise has been proposed to decrease production of these inflammatory agents, thus either increasing longevity, or increasing the duration of time we are able to maintain a physically active lifestyle. Regardless of the mechanism, though, it is well documented that people who maintain a high level of fitness have a decreased early mortality and in general a longer life without debilitating limitations.

Exercise and Its Role in Cancer Prevention and Survival

While the role of exercise in the prevention of cancer and the survival of cancer after diagnosis is a relatively new field, a great deal of research is currently being done in the area, with many promising results. Overall, exercise has been shown to reduce many cancers, particularly breast and colorectal cancers by as much as 20%–50%. Why does exercise and fitness decrease the risk of cancer? Its role in prevention of colon cancer is not yet fully understood, but it is generally thought that exercise and a high fiber diet speed up the movement of food through the large intestine. This decreases the amount of time that food (and possible carcinogens in the food) spends in contact with the tissue and may be the reason for the decreased risk of colorectal cancer. With breast cancer, the reasons are less understood, but exercise decreases some hormones, particularly insulin, and possibly estrogen-related hormones, and this may decrease the risk of breast cancer. Improvements in the immune response, which is seen with moderate intensity and duration exercise, may also be a factor in both types of cancer prevention. There is also some evidence that exercise decreases the risk of prostate and lung cancers, but this is not as clear as the evidence for the reduced risk of colon and breast cancer, and is confounded by other factors such as smoking (Emaus and Thune, 2011; Lee, 2003).

An even newer area of research is the role of exercise and fitness in the survival of cancer patients after they have been diagnosed and treated. Some studies indicate that people who are fit have an increased survival rate of at least several types of cancers, including colorectal, breast, and lung (Cleveland, et. al, 2012; Denlinger and Engstrom, 2011; Granger, et. al, 2011). Many possible reasons for the improved survival rate have been given that range from improved outlook on life (psychological), less muscle and heart atrophy from the treatments to improved immune responses, however, most are speculative at this point. The use of exercise in cancer rehabilitation is also an area in which research is increasing, so it is likely that mechanisms for the improved survival are likely to be found in the next few years.

Exercise Testing for Health and Fitness

You have covered the basics of exercise testing and training in the Clinical Exercise Physiology chapter. It is important, though, to distinguish between clinical and fitness testing. Remember the purposes of clinical exercise testing:

Diagnostic—to help determine the presence of disease.

Prognostic—to assess the likelihood of a positive outcome in a training program.

Functional—to evaluate the fitness status of the person.

In fitness testing, we have to make the assumption that the person we are testing is healthy and free of disease. Therefore, the purpose of fitness testing is solely functional in nature. For that reason, screening usually consists of the PAR-Q or a similar instrument that might be specific to the fitness facility. Screening may also include questions on lifestyle and on diet if that is one of the purposes of the facility. If, based on the screening tools, there is an indication of disease or increased risk factors, the client is usually referred to a clinical situation where appropriate medical supervision is available.

Fitness testing can range from simple field tests such as sit-ups and push-ups for muscle endurance and the one-mile walk for cardiorespiratory endurance to complicated and equipment-intensive maximal cycle or treadmill tests that actually measure Vo_2max. More often, tests are used that are relatively easy to interpret and help the fitness professional determine an exercise training regimen for the client. In this section we will describe some common tests for cardiorespiratory endurance, muscle strength, and muscle endurance that are used in many fitness settings.

Cardiorespiratory Endurance

Cardiorespiratory endurance (CRE) is the ability to perform exercise involving a large muscle mass for a prolonged period of time, usually ten or more minutes. The definition includes a large muscle mass because this requires the heart and lungs to work at a relatively high intensity to support the exercise and the duration requires aerobic metabolism, which also stresses the heart and lungs. CRE is usually tested using evaluations that last eight to twelve minutes and involve the legs, since they are the largest muscles in most people. The most common tests used worldwide are many of the field tests. One of the most common of these is the 1.5 mile run/walk. In this test, a flat area (a running track is one of the best) in which a 1.5 mile route can be set up is used. On a typical outdoor running track, this is six laps, but on indoor tracks this varies. The person or group is asked to run and walk as rapidly as they can to finish the 1.5 miles the fastest possible. The time it takes to complete 1.5 miles is recorded and compared to standard tables for an estimate of Vo_2max or fitness category. Figure 7–4 shows a graph of fitness category vs. time. There are also field tests involving one mile and 12 minutes, among others.

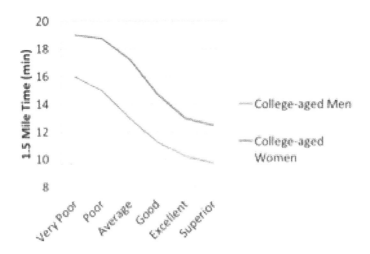

FIGURE 7-4. Graph of 1.5 mile finish time and fitness category for men and women ages 20–29.

Based on data from Cooper, K. *The Aerobics Program for Total Well-being*. Bantam Books, New York, 1982.

In addition to field tests, both submaximal and maximal laboratory tests can be performed to assess CRE. As with clinical exercise tests, these tests are typically performed on a treadmill or cycle ergometer, and may have oxygen uptake measured (Figure 7–5) or simply have it estimated by the load achieved during a maximal test, or by the heart rate and load performed during a submaximal test. As with the GXT in a clinical test, the speed and grade (treadmill) or load (cycle ergometer) is increased every one to three minutes until the subject cannot continue. At that point, the time and heart rate are noted or the V_{O_2} is noted and determined to be the maximal oxygen uptake.

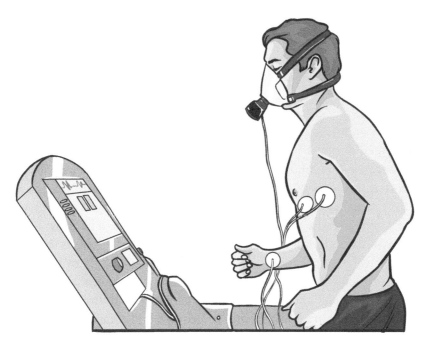

FIGURE 7-5. Example of a treadmill maximal test where V_{O_2} is being measured.

Muscle Strength and Endurance

Another major aspect of fitness is musculoskeletal strength and endurance. These are important factors in performance, but are also critical in elderly people as a means for maintaining the ability to perform normal daily activities. Muscle strength is defined as the maximal ability of a muscle or group of muscles to generate force, while muscle endurance is the ability to maintain or repeat submaximal contractions. Typical muscle strength measurements are done using weights or a dynamometer. This allows you to measure what is referred to as a 1-repetition maximum (1-RM). The 1-RM is the most weight (or force) that can be lifted one time. This is done by having the person lift a certain weight using a standard lift such as a bench press (see Figure 7–6). If the lift can be done, more weight is added until the lift cannot be accomplished. To be a valid test, it is generally suggested that the 1-RM be achieved within three to five attempts. As with other tests, the results of these are compared to normative values.

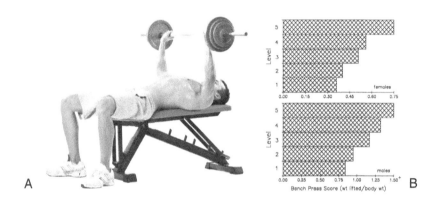

FIGURE 7–6. **A.** An example of a bench press. **B.** Normative values for bench press based on weight (Crouse and Coast, 2011).

© mihailomilovanovic, 2013. Used under license from Shutterstock, Inc. © Kendall Hunt Publishing

Tests of muscle endurance are typified by tests such as sit-ups or crunches, push-ups, and pull-ups or chin-ups (Figure 7–7). These need to be structured in a way, though, that the subject can do several—at least five—repetitions. If the person cannot do more than one or two repetitions, then the test is really a test of muscle strength, not endurance. As with the other tests, proper instructions need to be given, and when the test is completed it is often compared to norms. Sometimes values are not compared to norms, only to previous values achieved by the subject. This may be appropriate for a person who starts out in the lowest categories to help minimize embarrassment.

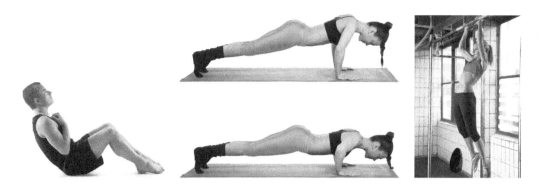

FIGURE 7–7. Examples of three muscular endurance tests: sit-ups, push-ups, and pull-ups.

© Lerche & Johnson, 2013. Used under license from Shutterstock, Inc. © dean bertoncelj, 2013. Used under license from Shutterstock, Inc. © Ammentorp Photography, 2013. Used under license from Shutterstock, Inc.

Body Composition

The estimation of body composition is another aspect of fitness testing. It can provide us information about the need (or lack thereof) for a subject to pursue weight loss. High levels of body fat are associated with increased risk of type 2 diabetes and heart disease and early mortality, so it is an important health measure as well. Ratios of height to weight, as in the measurement of body mass index (BMI) can provide a general estimate of whether a person is overweight or not, and high BMI values are often associated with overweight. However, in people with a lot of muscle mass, they are not accurate, so percent body fat is often estimated. Typical values of percent body fat for college-aged men and women are 13%–17% and 20%–25%, respectively. The measurement of body fatness has a lot of potential errors, but there are several estimates that give reasonably accurate results. Two common methods to estimate body fat are through underwater weighing and skinfolds (Figure 7–8). Long considered the "gold standard," underwater or hydrostatic weighing measures the density of the body, and uses that density to estimate body fat. This is based on the idea that fat is less dense (less mass per cubic centimeter) than muscle and bone so a person with less fat will weigh more when submerged in water than a person with more fat. A potential problem with this technique is that it is difficult to measure gas in the lungs, which has volume but almost no weight, so this contributes to errors in the measurement of density. Once an adequate level of proficiency in the measurement has been attained by the technician, most estimates using underwater weighing are with in 3%–5% of the true value. Another technique commonly used is the measurement of skinfold thickness. This technique assumes that a relatively constant portion of our fat is stored under the skin (i.e., subcutaneous). If we pinch the skin in places where people tend to store fat and in places where they do not, we can get an estimate of the subcutaneous fat and use that to estimate total fat. This technique is much less expensive than hydrostatic weighing, but also has errors, such as how hard the technician pulls the skinfolds. Typical measurements are within 5%–7% of true values. These techniques are widely used, and even if they have errors associated with them, we can easily say that if a person loses fat weight, these techniques should be able to detect it.

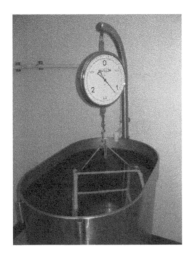
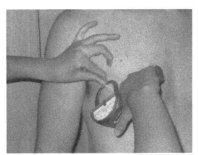

FIGURE 7–8. Two common techniques for estimating body fat, hydrostatic weighing, and skinfolds.

From *Clinical Exercise Physiology* by Stephen F. Crouse and J. Richard Coast. Copyright © 2011 by Kendall Hunt Publishing Company. Reprinted by permission.

Exercise Training for Fitness

We train for many reasons, including health, sport, or exercise performance and "good looks." You have seen the benefits of exercise and fitness from a health perspective, and we have discussed some of the results of training from a physiological viewpoint. Regardless of the reason for training, or even the method of training, the principles discussed in the Clinical Exercise Physiology chapter continue to be at play. That is, the body responds specifically to a system that is overloaded, in the manner to which it is overloaded. For example, if we overload the body with arm resistance exercise, the arms will get stronger and hypertrophy, but little or nothing happens to the legs. If we overload the body with endurance exercise, the cardiorespiratory system will respond by getting stronger and better able to deliver oxygen, and the muscles that are trained will respond by being better able to use the oxygen that is delivered, but our sprint ability is not likely to be improved. Further, if we stop training the adaptations are reversible; that is, we detrain. Also, people, while they tend to respond in a similar way, have individuality in their response. Some people tend to be better able to become strength athletes than others, and people have their own reasons for training, which may dictate how hard they work and what responses they gain. So the principles of training govern the responses in a healthy population as they do in a clinical population. In fact, you will likely note that we approach training for fitness in a very similar way to how we approach it in a clinical exercise prescription.

We structure our training based on the ideas of frequency, intensity, duration, and mode, or Frequency, Intensity, Time, and Type, the F.I.T.T. principle. This principle works whether we are setting up a resistance training program, an endurance training program, or a combination program designed primarily for overall fitness. Depending on what we desire from a training program, we can focus more on increasing intensity (for strength, speed, Vo_2max improvements) or on frequency and duration (muscular and cardiorespiratory endurance). Most training programs, though, increase all three aspects, but in differing amounts based on the goals of the training program. We will spend the rest of this section on some common methods to construct training programs for resistive and for dynamic training.

Resistance Training

The goal of a resistance training program for fitness and health is to increase muscle strength and endurance. This is an important type of training since as we age, muscle weakness is a tremendous hindrance to our ability to carry on acts of daily living. While there are nearly an infinite variety of individual training regimens for resistance training, most follow the principle of progressive resistive exercise. This principle incorporates periodic increases in intensity, duration, and frequency to provide an increasing level of stress to which the muscles must adapt. Intensity can be expressed as absolute weight (pounds or kilograms), as a percent of body weight, or as a percent of the 1-RM. Duration is the number of sets and repetitions (reps) that are completed in a workout. There are usually more sets and reps when the weight is low and fewer when the weight is near the 1-RM. Frequency is the number of times per week that the exercise is performed.

For general fitness, a typical starting resistance training regimen consists of two to three sets of eight to ten reps with 60%–80% 1-RM as the intensity. Usually exercises are divided by days with two days set aside for lower body and two for upper body, each with five to seven different exercises. It is probably more common, though, for people with time constraints to exercise two to three days per week with a total of eight to ten exercises, divided between upper and lower body.

For athletes, a much more structured approach is taken to resistance training. Power athletes and Olympic-style weight lifters, for whom both strength and speed are extremely important usually do fewer repetitions (three to eight) with much more weight, while endurance athletes typically perform more repetitions (10–15, or even 20) with less weight. There are also what are termed periodization schedules that are often set up for strength athletes in weight training. Periodization involves a series of micro-, meso-, and macrocycles around which the intensity, sets, and reps are changed on a time schedule of one to four weeks. This change in program is not simply a periodic increase in weights, sets or reps, but a combination of increases and decreases in these. For example, as intensity is increased during one cycle, the number of sets and reps might be decreased slightly to allow the athlete to accommodate and gain strength. Keep in mind the principle of specificity, if the desire is to increase strength maximally, then an increase in weight is required. When this happens, the number of repetitions that the athlete can perform must be decreased.

Dynamic Training

Dynamic training traditionally consists of moving the body through space with little more resistance than the weight of the body. However, some of the pieces of exercise equipment seen in fitness facilities simulate the movements without actually having the person move anywhere (Figure 7–9). Dynamic exercise can be performed in many situations, specific to the metabolic system that is being trained. For example, if you run maximally for 30 seconds, or jog for 20 minutes, the activity is similar, but the results will be very different. Why?

Aerobic training is what we think of usually in fitness and health related dynamic training. This type of training is done at a submaximal pace and usually lasts 15–20 minutes or longer. The standard advice given by many books and fitness professionals is that we need to train 20–30 minutes per day (duration) for three to five days per week (frequency) at a pace that requires 60%–80%

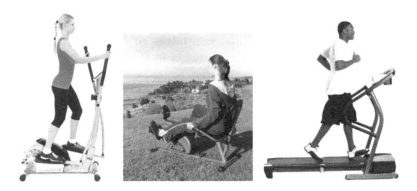

FIGURE 7-9. Equipment that allows us to perform dynamic exercise training without moving through space, an elliptical trainer, a recumbent cycle ergometer, and a treadmill.

© Serghei Starus, 2013. Used under license from Shutterstock, Inc. © Neo Edmund, 2013. Used under license from Shutterstock, Inc. © Flashon Studio, 2013. Used under license from Shutterstock, Inc.

of Vo_2max (intensity). As with resistance training, though, there are a nearly infinite combination of frequencies, intensities, and durations that are possible that can still be effective. Some new evidence, for example, suggests that several bouts of exercise of five to ten minutes duration are as good as one 20–30 minute bout, particularly for sedentary people. It should be obvious that endurance athletes need much more exercise than do people training for basic health and fitness, but there is a trade-off. As the intensity, duration, and frequency increase, so does the incidence of injury. For health and fitness, we desire to achieve the gains in fitness, as expressed by an improvement in Vo_2max, without increasing our injury risk. Athletes, however, have to exercise to achieve performance gains that are maximized, and have to assume the risks of increased injury (Figure 7–10).

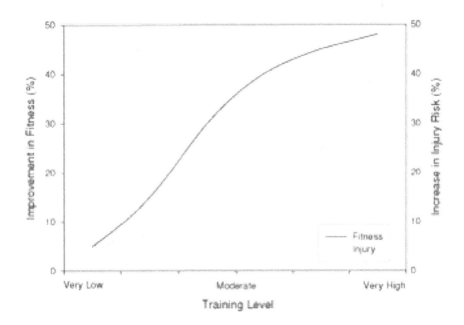

FIGURE 7-10. Diagram of the trade-off between the improvements in fitness and the increases in injury risk with increased levels of training.

One good way to monitor training intensity is through heart rate. The typical training zone of 60%–80% Vo_2max elicits a heart rate of approximately 70%–90% of maximal heart rate. We think of this as a good training zone for improvements in Vo_2max, although different people respond differently and some require a higher or lower heart rate. Remember that one of the major adaptations to endurance training is a lower heart rate at rest and at submaximal exercise. As we train, then, it requires more intense exercise to achieve the same heart rate, so by monitoring heart rate we not only maintain a proper intensity, but we achieve a good progression involving the ten percent rule.

We also use anaerobic training in some cases. This would be accomplished by performing short bursts of exercise at or near maximal levels, followed by rest or by exercise of lower intensity. We refer to this as interval training. Interval training is usually used mainly by athletes specifically training for power or speed events.

Exercise and Sport Nutrition

While nutrition is a field in itself, it merits inclusion in a chapter on health, fitness, and wellness since proper nutrition is a key ingredient in health and wellness. From a fitness and exercise perspective, adequate and appropriate nutrition is an extremely important factor in performance. Just as there is a great deal of misinformation in the exercise field, so is there a lot of incorrect material in nutrition and diets that are proposed just to sell products. This section will not concentrate on the misinformation, but rather on helping you understand what is proper nutrition and what may need to be done to the diet to enhance health and performance.

Nutrients are divided into three types, macronutrients, micronutrients, and water, although water is not always given its own category. Macronutrients are those that compose a large part of a healthy diet and are used as fuels and for structure. These include fats, carbohydrates, and proteins. Micronutrients compose relatively small parts of a healthy diet, and usually work with the macronutrients to help the body function properly. They consist of vitamins and minerals. Then water, of course, is vitally important. It does not make up any of the calorie content of the diet, but composes over 70% of our mass, so it is critical to keep these stores at adequate levels. While we can survive for days to weeks without adequate levels of certain micronutrients, and can fast for several days before suffering decrements in our daily lives due to lack of macronutrients, we can lose enough water in just a few days to cause death, so it is very important in a healthy diet.

Macronutrients

Carbohydrates

Carbohydrates are chemical compounds composed only of carbon, hydrogen, and oxygen. In exercise, carbohydrates make up the majority of the fuel we use in most cases. The complete breakdown of one gram of carbohydrates provides approximately four kilocalories of energy. If we use carbohydrates as fuel, we get approximately 5.0 kcal of energy for every liter of oxygen we consume. Carbohydrates consist of simple sugars or monosaccharides such as glucose and fructose. There are also disaccharides, or combinations of two simple sugars. Sucrose or table sugar is one of the most familiar, and consists of one glucose and one fructose molecule. Finally there are the polysaccharides or complex carbohydrates. These consist of chains of glucose and are the storage form of carbohydrates. Starch and glycogen are the two primary polysaccharides. Starch is found in plants, while glycogen is the storage form of carbohydrate in animals.

The breakdown of carbohydrates occurs in the body in the metabolic pathways consisting of glycolysis, the Krebs or citric acid cycle, and the electron transport system (for a review of these systems, see Chapter 2). Carbohydrates are readily used as fuel, and compose the majority (up to 100%) of the energy used for exercise tasks lasting up to one an hour, particularly relatively intense tasks. Most of this comes from glycogen in the muscles, but some comes from blood glucose and some from supplements taken during the exercise itself. Most nutritionists suggest that approximately 60% of the calories in our diet come from carbohydrates, with most of that coming from complex carbohydrates, such as whole grains.

Fats

Fats, also referred to as lipids, are critical nutrients, even though they generally have a bad reputation in the diet world. It is the major storage form of energy in the body, with approximately 20–40 times the amount kilocalories stored as fat, compared to that stored as glycogen. We get approximately nine kilocalories from burning one gram of fat. If we use fat as a fuel during exercise we get approximately 4.7 kcal for each liter of oxygen consumed. In a person of average weight, there is enough fat to allow them to walk 70+ hours without running out of fat energy. Fats are also critical for protection of internal organs and for the formation and transport of the lipid soluble vitamins—A, D, E, and K.

While fats are found in numerous forms in the body, including in cell membranes, the primary form in which they occur, and which is the form that they are stored, is called triglyceride. This consists of one glycerol (a three carbon carbohydrate) molecule with three fatty acids attached to it. These fatty acids yield most of the energy when broken down. They are metabolized in β-oxidation, the Krebs cycle, and the electron transport system. These fatty acids vary in length from about 12 to about 20 carbons long and are classified by how many of the binding sites on the carbon chains are filled (or saturated) with hydrogens. A carbon chain where all available sites are bound by hydrogen molecules is said to be saturated. If one site does not have a hydrogen bound to it, that fatty acid is monounsaturated. If more than one site is unbound with hydrogen, it is polyunsaturated. Most animal fats, as well as palm and coconut oils are saturated. Olive and canola oils are monounsaturated fats, while corn and peanut oils are polyunsaturated. There is evidence that the unsaturated fats are more healthy and may lead to lower risk of cardiovascular disease. Saturated fats are associated with increases in cardiovascular disease, as well as possibly colon and breast cancers. Nutritionists suggest that total fat intake, regardless of the type of fat, should be less than approximately 30% of the calories, with 10% or less coming from saturated fats.

Proteins

These are the third macronutrient category. Proteins are chains of amino acids. While proteins can be used for energy, their major purpose is structure and in control of bodily functions. They compose a large portion of muscle, as well as part of the cell membranes. Many enzymes, which catalyze reactions in the body, such as those for metabolism, are protein based as well. Many of the hormones that control cellular and tissue function also consist of proteins, so their importance is very high.

Generally it is recommended that protein form 10%–15% of the caloric content of the diet. Excess protein consumption can lead in some people to increases in liver and kidney damage. The recommendation for protein in the diet translates to approximately one gram protein per kilogram body weight per day. The increases in protein that might be needed by an athlete are thought to be covered by the increase in the total diet. That is, if an athlete needs 50% more calories, yet maintains a protein content of 10%–15% of the diet, then he or she will supply all the extra protein that is needed, and there is no need for an athlete to specifically supplement with protein. Some studies suggest, though, that in the early stages of a training program, or when an athlete suddenly increases the volume of training, there may be a need to take in a few percent more protein for the first one to two weeks, when there may be an amino acid deficit.

Micronutrients

Vitamins

Vitamins are organic compounds that are required for certain bodily functions, but which cannot be synthesized within the body. They are very important in energy metabolism and in other functions such as helping form bone, but they cannot be used as fuels or as structural components themselves. There are two categories of vitamins, fat soluble and water soluble. The fat soluble vitamins are A, D, E, and K, while the water soluble vitamins are the group of B vitamins and vitamin C.

The requirement for vitamins is generally very small, and either too little or too much can cause health problems. For example, a lack of vitamin D, which we get from fish and eggs, as well as fortified milk, causes a bone disease called rickets, which is a softening of the bones, sometimes leading to deformed bones (an example is bow-leggedness). However, too much vitamin intake can lead to toxicity in some cases. This is particularly true of the fat soluble vitamins, which are stored in the liver and other organs. While the water soluble vitamins can be toxic, this is usually less of a problem since they are more easily excreted in the urine.

Most people have adequate vitamins assuming they eat a balanced diet. Some people do have vitamin deficiencies and these can be diagnosed by a physician. Most nutritionists and health experts suggest that there is no need to supplement with vitamins unless there is a documented deficiency. As with protein, athletes are not generally thought to need supplements of vitamins, since the possible increased need should be met by the increased food intake required for the extra calories required.

Minerals

These are inorganic substances that are used to assist enzymes, form bones, and other activities such as clotting and carrying impulses through the nerves and muscles. Calcium and phosphorus are important in bone formation. Sodium, potassium, and chloride ions are important in nerve and muscle transmission of impulses. As with vitamins, most minerals can be obtained in an adequate diet. Women may have an increased need for iron and calcium, though.

Water

Water is, indeed, the "stuff of life." It is required for virtually all cell functions. In exercise, water replenishment is critically important. We use it, in the form of evaporation of perspiration, to cool our bodies during exercise or on a warm/hot day. In this process, we can lose over a liter of fluid per hour during even moderate intensity exercise in a warm environment. Replenishment is critical to performance, and even to survival. For example, dehydration is one of the major causes of death and illness to hikers in the Grand Canyon.

The issue of dehydration during exercise has led to an entire industry in sports beverages. For the majority of our exercise needs, water is sufficient. Prolonged exercise (more than one to two hours), particularly in a hot environment, leads to a loss of minerals as well as water, so many people have devised fluid replacement beverages. These beverages often include sodium and potassium, as well as various formulations of carbohydrates. Many studies have shown that certain of these beverages improve performance in long-duration exercise when compared to water. Others have evaluated the beverages and argue that they have too high of a concentration of minerals and sugars, which may lead to a decrease in the ability of the fluid to empty from the intestine and actually replace lost water in the body. General guidelines for fluid replacement drinks are to have them cool, with low concentrations of minerals and other solids (like carbohydrates) and make them palatable. These guidelines appear to result in a fluid that replaces the lost fluid, some of the minerals and carbohydrates that are lost, and will be consumed in adequate amounts by the athlete.

There are almost as many diets designed for exercise as there are people who exercise, but there is no real secret to exercise nutrition. Most sport nutritionists agree, though, that a balanced diet that meets the caloric requirements of the athlete is the most desirable. Some athletes find that they perform better with a particular diet than with another and that certain dietary practices prior to competition help them. Whether the specific diet that a person uses is the best one is highly debatable, but it is probably good for an athlete to consume a diet that is consistent with what is normally consumed and is palatable to keep from having gastrointestinal problems associated with a novel consumption of food that may not be agreeable.

Exercise Myths

Along with the good things that come with exercise, there have been many fads and a lot of misinformation in the exercise field. Many of these come with weight loss and its associated exercise and diet regimens. At best, these are incorrect, but they may go beyond being wrong and in some cases actually harm the person performing them. One of the difficult aspects of these myths is that they often start with a valid point then take that point to a level that is not realistic. Let's go through a few common exercise fads and misconceptions.

Lactic Acid Causes Muscle Soreness

This is a tough question, because it is so prevalant in the fitness industry. Who hasn't heard from a coach, trainer, or fitness "guru" that lactic acid causes muscle soreness and that if we can decrease the production or increase the removal of lactic acid our muscles will not get sore? The idea is an easy one to grasp and was originally proposed more than 80 years ago; after all, if you put a drop of vinegar (acetic acid) on a scratch, it stings, so that makes it easy to see why that might be the case with muscle soreness. There are two types of muscle soreness: 1) acute soreness, which occurs during or immediately following exercise; and 2) delayed soreness, which starts about 24–48 hours after exercise and lasts for about two to four days. Acute soreness is generally thought to be related to ischemia or lack of blood flow, and may be related to acid accumulation, including lactic acid. Acute soreness goes away immediately or within a few minutes after you stop exercising. Delayed soreness appears to have nothing to do with lactic acid. The first line of evidence for this conclusion is that the lactic acid is completely back to resting levels within 15–30 minutes after exercise. Research starting in the 1970's has shown that this type of soreness is caused by damage to the muscles and the resulting inflammation, which stimulates pain receptors in the muscle. Many suggestions have been made to deal with soreness, from exercise to massage to anti-inflammatory drugs such as aspirin or ibuprofen, but none of these seem to have more than temporary effects.

Spot Reduction

The idea behind spot reduction is that you lose fat in areas that you exercise, so if you have a lot of "belly fat" then sit-ups, crunches, or other exercises in the abdominal area will cause you to lose fat there (Figure 7–11). This is a favorite tool of late night infomercials and fitness magazines. A recent study (Kostek, et. al, 2007) actually looked at MRI images to show that arm exercise doesn't cause spot reduction in fat. What most of the carefully conducted studies have shown is that by creating a caloric deficit (more calories expended than taken in) we mobilize fat through the whole body through hormone actions. When this happens fat decreases all around the body, and where would you expect to see the most fat loss? That's correct, most of the fat is lost from where most is deposited, and if most is deposited around the waist, most will be lost there. The same resulting fat loss would happen in a running or cycling program as well, just as long as we create a caloric deficit through exercise and diet. What may happen in some cases that claim to show a reduction in waist circumference is toning of the muscles. That is, most people who have a lot of fat in the waist area also have weak abdominal and back muscles, resulting in a protrusion (sticking out) of the abdomen. As the muscles become toned, through core exercises such as sit-ups, people are better able to hold the abdomen in toward the body and this results in a decrease in waist circumference.

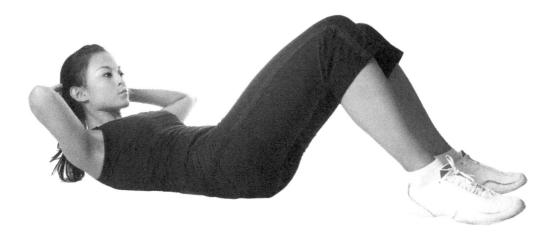

FIGURE 7–11. Sit-ups do not cause a specific reduction in abdominal fat.
© Jurjah Mosin, 2013. Used under license from Shutterstock, Inc.

Long, Slow Exercise Burns Fat Better

This is a popular myth that comes up very often and has its roots in well-done scientific studies, but has been misinterpreted. The Respiratory Exchange Ratio (RER) that was described in Chapter 2 allows us to determine whether fats or carbohydrates are used as a fuel, either at rest or during exercise. Numerous studies, dating back nearly 100 years, have shown that at low intensities we tend to burn more fat, and as exercise duration increases we tend to use a higher proportion of fat than we do during short-duration, high-intensity exercise. This has been misinterpreted by many to suggest that as the way to lose fat weight. The reality is that weight gain or loss is simply a matter of calories taken in vs. calories expended, NOT the fuel we use during exercise. In order to lose weight, one must "burn" more calories than he takes in. Weight loss is best accomplished by a simultaneous reduction in food intake with an increase in exercise. There are other reasons, though, why someone might want to use low-intensity exercise, such as balance issues associated with age, obesity, or neural disability, or a lack of fitness that requires using low-intensity exercise at the beginning of an exercise regimen, but fat loss is not one of the reasons.

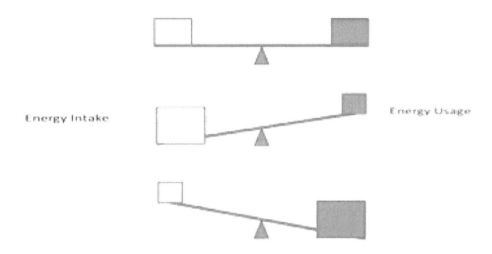

Energy Intake   Energy Usage

FIGURE 7–12. Weight loss is accomplished by expending more calories than one takes in. The top scale shows energy intake and usage equal, no weight gain or loss; the middle scale shows intake larger than usage, weight gain; the bottom scale shows usage greater than intake, weight loss. The balance of fat vs carbohydrate used during exercise is much less important.

Muscle Burns Two or Five, or Ten, or Twenty Times the Calories than Fat Does, So if You Gain Muscle You Can Lose Fat During Your Sleep or at Rest, or While at Your Desk

This is another popular myth that is stated as fact in many fitness and health magazines. The claim is that by doing resistance exercise, you gain muscle mass, and muscle mass has a much greater metabolic rate than fat or other tissues. Therefore, by gaining muscle mass, you increase your metabolic rate, even when resting or doing quiet work, such as studying, thereby losing weight "while you sleep." Skeletal muscle has a tremendous advantage, in that it can increase its metabolic rate from rest to exercise by hundreds of times. However, at rest the metabolic rate of fat (~12 kJ/kg body weight/day) and muscle (~25–60 kJ/kg/day) only differ by about two to four times. The real energy users at rest are the liver (~1000 kJ/kg/day), brain (~1000 kJ/kg/day), and kidneys (~2000 kJ/kg/day), which use energy at a rate 15–30 times higher than muscle (Illner, et. al, 2000; Nelson, et. al, 1992).

So, the question comes down to what would happen if we replaced a certain amount of fat with muscle; let's explore that. If we gained 4 kg (~10 lbs) of muscle—which is difficult to do, that would increase our energy expenditure by 100–240 kJ/day (4kg X 25 kJ/kg/day to 4 kg X 60 kJ/kg/day) or approximately 36,500 to 87,600 per year. This is sufficient to lose 2.5 to 6.0 pounds of fat (1 pound of fat = about 14,600 kJ). That is not bad, but certainly not the amount of increased metabolic rate that the fitness magazines describe, and don't forget that in replacing this fat with muscle, we have lost 4 kg of fat which would have burned about 48 kJ/day (4 kg X 12 kJ/kg/day) or 17,500 kJ/year or about 1.25 pounds of fat. Therefore, replacing fat with muscle will increase weight loss, but the effect is relatively small. It is still critical to exercise in order to increase the metabolic rate of the muscle and expend energy during exercise.

You Expend More Energy Lifting Weights Since It Is So Intense

Another "fact" proposed by some fitness professionals and magazines is that since you work so hard and your muscles "burn" during weight lifting, you are burning a lot of energy, even more than during aerobic exercise. There is no question that weight lifting can be very intense, and even painful. Studies indicate that the Vo_2 during squat and bench press exercises can be as high as 2–3 L/min (Roberts, et. al, 2007). This compares well with jogging or cycling, where jogging at 10 min/mile for a 70 kg (~155 pound) person would use about 2.5 L/min of oxygen. Keep in mind, though, that during resistance training, actual lifting of weights and expending of energy only takes place about ½ the time, with the other ½ of the time taking place as recovery. Therefore, while resistance training is a very important component of a general fitness program, and critical for power sports, its effect on metabolism is not as great as is aerobic exercise.

So, Why, if Resistance Training Does Not Cause a Person to Expend Such a Great Amount of Energy That It Is a Great Weight Loss Technique, Do I See Such "Ripped" People in the Fitness Magazines?

Great question, and the answer may be different for different people or animals. In some cases it is genetic, while in other cases, they have worked very hard (or used other means) to achieve the degree of hypertrophy that allows muscles to be seen under the skin. In addition, most have very low amounts of body fat in the subcutaneous area, thus making it easier to see the muscles. This very low body fat is generally accomplished by both a lot of heavy exercise and a diet that achieves a caloric deficit sufficient to decrease the subcutaneous fat to the extent needed.

The point of this section on exercise myths is not to describe each one, nor is it to indicate that all the information in fitness magazines or given by fitness professionals is full of errors. What one needs to do, though, after reading or listening to these types of claims is to examine them. Go to the textbooks, research and scientific literature before you believe that Substance X will cause you to lose weight, gain muscle, and generally become more attractive.

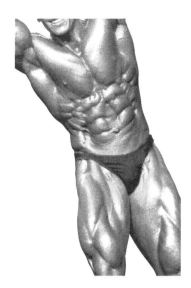
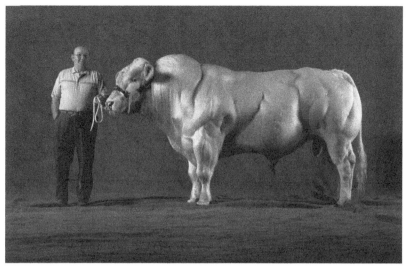

FIGURE 7–13. Two examples of "ripped" muscles.

© Gabi Moisa, 2013. Used under license from Shutterstock, Inc. © Yann Arthus-Bertrand/Corbis.

Glossary

1-RM—One-repetition maximum. The highest amount of weight that can be lifted in one exercise.

Cardiorespiratory endurance—The ability of the body to conduct large muscle mass exercise for a period of time.

Disaccharide—A carbohydrate composed of two simple sugars.

Fitness—The ability to carry on activities that are expected of a person. Usually refers to physical health.

Health—The absence of disease. Usually a combination of physical fitness and mental health.

Hydrostatic Weighing—A method of estimating body composition using underwater weight.

Interval Training—A type of exercise training that involves periods of relatively high intensity exercise followed by periods of rest or relatively low intensity exercise.

Macronutrient—The components of a diet consumed in large amounts for fuel or structure. Consist of carbohydrates, lipids, and proteins.

Micronutrient—The components of a diet consumed in very small amounts to supplement the activities of bodily processes. Consist of vitamins and minerals.

Monosaccharide—Another term for a simple sugar.

Muscle Endurance—The ability of a muscle or group of muscles to sustain a submaximal force or repeated submaximal contractions over time.

Muscle Strength—The ability of a muscle or group of muscles to generate a maximal force.

Polysaccharide—A long chain of simple sugars. Consist of starch and glycogen.

Saturated Fatty Acid—A lipid chain in which all of the binding sites on the carbon atoms are occupied by a hydrogen atom.

Skinfold Technique—Method of estimating body composition using the thickness of skinfolds to measure subcutaneous fat stores.

Unsaturated Fatty Acid—A lipid chain in which some of the binding sites on the carbon atoms are not occupied by a hydrogen atom.

Wellness—An overarching term of health that encompasses physical, social, intellectual, mental, environmental, and spiritual health.

General References

Dunford, M. 2010. *Fundamentals of Sport and Exercise Nutrition.* Champaign, IL: Human Kinetics.

Edlin, G. and E. Golanty. 1992. *Health and Wellness. A Holistic Approach.* Boston: Jones and Bartless Publishers.

Powers, S. K., S. L. Dodd, and E. M. Jackson. 2011. *Total Fitness and Wellness,* 5 ed. Boston: Benjamin Cummings.

Ratamess, N. *ACSM's 2012. Foundations of Strength Training and Conditioning.* Philadelphia: Lippincott Williams and Wilkins.

References to Specific Studies

Arias, E. 2004. "United States Life Tables, National Vital Statistice Reports." *Centers for Disease Control* (53) Number 6.

Blair, S. N., H. W. Kohl III, R. S. Paffenbarger, D. G. Clark, K. H. Cooper, and L. W. Gibbons. 1989. "Physical Fitness and All-cause Mortality: A Prospective Study of Healthy Men and Women." *J. Am. Med. Assoc.* 262:2395–2401.

Carter, C. S., T. Hofer, A. Y. Seo, and C. Leeuwenburgh. 2007. "Molecular Mechanisms of Life- and Health-span Extension: Role of Calorie Restriction and Exercise Intervention." *Appl. Physiol. Nutr. Metab.* 32:954–66.

Castelli, W. P. 1988. "Cholesterol and Lipids in the Risk of Coronary Artery Disease—The Framingham Heart Study." *Can. J. Cardiol.* 4(Suppl A):5A–10A.

Cleveland, R. J., S. M. Eng, J. Stevens, P. T. Bradshaw, S. L. Teitelbaum, A. I. Neugut, and M. D. Gammon. 2012. "Influence of Prediagnostic Recreational Physical Activity on Survival from Breast Cancer." *Eur. J. Cancer Prev.* 21:46–54.

Denlinger, C. S. and P. F. Bergstrom. 2011. "Colorectal Cancer Survivorship: Movement Matters." *Cancer Prev. Res.* 4:502–11.

Emaus, A. and I. Thune. 2011. "Physical Activity and Lung Cancer Prevention." *Rec. Results Cancer Res.* 186:101–33.

Fox, C. S., N. P. Paynter, M. J. Pencina, R. S. Vasan, P. W. F. Wilson, and R. B. D'Agostino. 2008. "Lifetime Risk of Cardiovascular Disease With and Without Diabetes Stratified by Obesity Status in the Framingham Heart Study." *Diabetes Care* 31:1582–84.

Granger, C. L., C. F. McDonald, S. Berney, C. Chao, and L. Denehy. 2011. "Exercise Intervention to Improve Exercise Capacity and Health Related Quality of Life for Patients with Non-small Cell Lung Cancer: A Systematic Review." *Lung Cancer* 72:139–53.

Hubert, H. B., M. Feinleib, P. M. McNamara, and W. P. Castelli. 1983. "Obesity as an Independent Risk Factor for Cardiovascular Disease: A 26-year Follow-up of Participants in the Framingham Heart Study." *Circulation* 67:968–77.

Illner, K., G. Brinkmann, M. Heller, A. Bosy-Westphal, and M.J. Müller. 2000. "Metabolically Active Components of Fat Free Mass and Resting Energy Expenditure in Nonobese Adults." *Am. J. Physiol.* 278:E308–E315.

Kostek, M. A., L. S. Pescatello, R. L. Seip, T. J. Angelopoulos, P. M. Clarkson, P. M. Gordon, N. M. Moyna, et. al. 2007. "Subcutaneous Fat Alterations Resulting from an Upper-body Resistance Training Program." *Med. Sci. Sports Exerc.* 39:1177–85.

Lee, I. M. 2003. "Physical Activity and Cancer Prevention—Data from Epidemiological Studies." *Med. Sci. Sports Exerc.* 35:1823–27.

Levitsky, Y. S., M. J. Pencina, R. B. D'Agostino, J. B. Meigs, J. M. Murabito, R. S. Vasan, and C. S. Fox. 2008. "Impact of Impaired Fasting Glucose on Cardiovascular Disease." The Framingham Heart Study. *J. Am. Coll. Cardiol.* 51:264–70.

Miles, W. P. and P. M. Clarkson. 1994. "Exercise-induced Muscle Pain, Soreness, and Cramps." *J Sports Med Phys Fitness* 34:203–16.

Morris, J. N., S. P. W. Chave, C. Adam, C. Sirey, L. Epstein, and D. J. Sheehan. 1973. "Vigorous Exercise in Leisure-time: Protection Against Coronary Heart-disease." *Lancet* 1:333–39.

Muller, F. L., M. S. Lustgarten, Y. Jang, A. Richardson, and H. Van Remmen. 2007. "Trends in Oxidative Aging Theories." *Free Rad. Biol. and Med.* 43:477–503.

Nelson, K. M., R. L. Weinsier, C. L. Long, and Y Schutz. 1992. "Predition of Resting Energy Expenditure from Fat-free Mass and Fat Mass." *Am. J. Clin. Nutr.* 56:848–56.

Robergs, R. A., T. Gordon, J. Reynolds, and T. B. Walker. 2007. "Energy Expenditure During Bench Press and Squat Exercises." *J. Str. Cond. Res.* 21:123–30.

Chapter 8
SPORTS PSYCHOLOGY

Although the field of psychology is centuries old, the application of psychology to sports as an academic discipline is relatively new, extending back only about 100 years. According to the American Psychological Association, psychology is the study of mind and behavior. Sports psychology has been defined as "the application of psychological theory and methods to the understanding and enhancement of athletic performance" (Kremer and Moran, 2008). Within sports psychology we can ask two fundamental questions, which are ultimately circular: How does psychology affect sports (or exercise) behavior? And, does sports (or exercise) participation affect the participant's psychology?

History

The idea that exercise is good for both physical and mental health is not new. This belief was held firmly by Frenchman Pierre de Coubertin (1863–1937) and was one of the factors motivating him to found the International Olympic Committee (IOC) in 1894. Coubertin was keenly interested in the application of psychology to athletes, and in 1900 published a text called simply "La psychologic du sport." In this text, Coubertin lamented that research in sports psychology lagged far behind research in physiology (Kornspan, 2007). Prominent educators in the United States shared Coubertin's belief that exercise was good for the body and mind. In 1859, Reverend William Augustus Stearn (1805–1876), President of Amherst College in Massachusetts, endorsed regular exercise as good for his students' well-being and academic success. He said that "If a moderate amount of physical exercise could be secured as a general thing to every student daily, I have a deep conviction . . . that not only would lives and health be preserved but animation and cheerfulness and a higher order of efficient study and intellectual life would be secured" (Marsh, 1952). Despite the sentiment that exercise is good for health and character, at that time, as Coubertin noted, research on sport psychology was limited. One of the first studies in sports psychology *per se* was published by Triplett in 1898 on a phenomenon known as social facilitation. In this study, competitive cyclists were tested in three scenarios—a time trial in which the cyclist raced along on a track, a paced time trial in which the cyclist was paced by another cyclist, and head-to-head competition. The cyclists were fastest in the competition trials, leading Triplett to conclude that " . . . the bodily presence of another contestant participating simultaneously in the race serves to liberate latent energy not ordinarily found" (Triplett, 1898). We'll return to this observation when we discuss group dynamics.

Coleman Robert Griffith (1893–1966) is credited as being the "father of American sports psychology." His 1925 paper entitled "Psychology and its Relation to Athletic Competition" pointed out what we now take as obvious—that psychological factors affect athletes and athletic performance. Griffith inaugurated the Athletic Research Laboratory at the University of Illinois, and served as its director from 1925 until the laboratory closed in the wake of the Great Depression in 1932. Research conducted in the laboratory included studies on psychomotor skills (like reaction time), learning, and personality. Griffith corresponded with football stars such as Knut Rockne, legendary coach of Notre Dame, and Red Grange, a running back who became a college and professional Hall of Fame member. However, Griffith's best known foray into popular sports was with the Chicago Cubs. By 1937, owner Philip Wrigley was frustrated by the decline of his team, which had made it to (but lost) the World Series in 1932 and 1935. Wrigley hired Griffith to apply psychological principles to his team, probably the first time a professional team employed a sports psychologist. Griffith started with the Cubs at their spring training in 1938, and continued until 1940. He and his assistant made many observations and provided Wrigley with numerous recommendations, essentially none of which were implemented. The Cub's manager, Charlie Grimm, was likely obstructionist, and not all players were receptive to a person Grimm told them was a "headshrinker."

After the closure of the Griffith laboratory, sports psychology research in the United States underwent a long drought until a revival in the 1960's. The North American Society for the Psychology of Sport and Physical Activity (NASPSPA) was founded in 1967, the Journal of Sports Psychology in 1970, and the Association for Applied Sports Psychology was created in 1986. In 1988, the US Olympic team included a sports psychologist for the first time (Kremer and Moran, 2008).

Personality

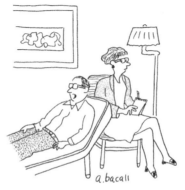

"I have multiple personalities and they are all following me on Twitter."

FIGURE 8-1. Cartoon on personality.

www.CartoonStock.com

Personality is an everyday term. We've all tried at some point to describe someone else's personality, or our own. But what exactly is personality? The American Psychological Society defines personality as "the unique psychological qualities of an individual that influence a variety of characteristic behavior patterns." How do we know or judge personality? When you see a handsome stranger from across a crowded room, you may immediately start to form ideas about that individual's personality. On what evidence are those ideas based? When evaluating recruits or potential draftees, coaches and owners are interested in personality. Are there personality traits that can predict athletic success? Particularly when we consider children, we may also want to know if sports participation can influence personality. These are some of the interesting questions addressed in personality research.

Assignment 8–1.　Write a description of your own personality using at least 15 words or short phrases. Do not use complete sentences. Have a roommate or friend do the same—describe your personality in 15 words or short phrases. How much overlap is there? Does your friend perceive you as you perceive yourself?

Personality psychology is a field replete with theories. Textbooks on personality typically cover a dozen or more theories, usually centered around the individual who created and promoted the idea. For example, nearly all personality textbooks have a chapter dedicated to Sigmund Freud (1856–1939) and his psychoanalytic approach to personality. For our purposes, we'll cover two *types* of personality theories, those that are deterministic and those that fall under the realm of social learning theory. Deterministic models of personality assume that personality has a stable biological basis. According to this perspective, personality is rooted in genetics and physiology, and is little influenced by the environment or experience. Psychoanalysts such as Freud and Carl Jung (1875–1961) postulated this type of model. Social learning theories put more emphasis on the environment and experiences in shaping the personality of the individual.

One of the oldest deterministic concepts of temperament, if not personality, is the "humors" model of the ancient Greeks. They believed that personality is based on four bodily humors: blood, bile, black bile, and phlegm. According to this idea, optimism and happiness are related to blood. The English word "sanguine" comes from this connection. A person who is tense and easy to anger is choleric, related to bile. Black bile (which doesn't really exist) makes a person melancholy, or pessimistic and sad. Finally, phlegm is related to being calm, dull, and slow. You might assume that these ideas were deserted few centuries ago, but not so—you can still find references to these four dimensions in modern discussions of personality. For example, in a series of articles on leadership, author David Lykken, a mortgage banker and radio personality, used the four categories of sanguine, choleric, melancholic, and phlegmatic to characterize peoples' personalities (Figure 8–2). According to Mr. Lykken (2011), "How well we relate and communicate with each other has as much to do with our personality types as anything, and therefore, it is essential . . . to incorporate a thorough understanding of these four personality types in our day-to-day communication."

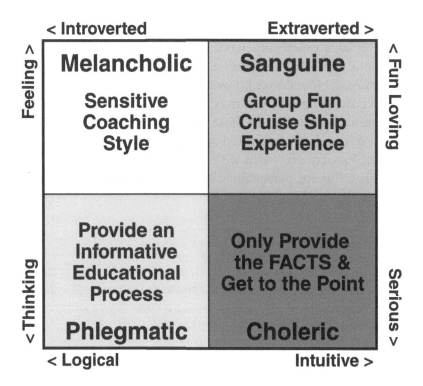

FIGURE 8–2. Personality categories following the ancient Greek model. David Lykken 2/28/11 http://nationalmortgageprofessional.com/news23841/are-you-relatable

From: *Are You Relatable?* By David Lykken. Http://nationalmortgageprofessional.com/news23841/are-you-relatable. Reprinted by permission of NMP Media Corp.

The Greek humors model of temperament is essentially a "trait" model—a construction based on biological personality traits. Elements of this ancient construct are reflected in the original two-factor personality model created by Hans Eysenck (1916–1997, pronounced "eye-sink"). Eysenck used a powerful statistical tool called factor analysis to identify two fundamental "dimensions" of personality which he called extraversion and neuroticism (Eysenck, 1947). Extraversion is the tendency to seek stimulation and gratification outside of the self. Its opposite is introversion. Neuroticism is the tendency toward anxiety and vulnerability to stress. Its opposite is mental stability. Twenty-nine years later, Eysenck and his collaborator (his wife) added a third factor called psychoticism. Psychoticism is the tendency toward recklessness, hostility, low social sensitivity, and non-conformist behavior (Howarth, 1986). The three factors together are known as the PEN model of personality. Eysenck's model is deterministic; he believed that these global personality traits are based on physiology, for example, psychoticism is related to testosterone levels, and in fact males tend to score higher on this scale.

Eysenck was not the only psychologist to develop a traits-based model of personality. Contemporaneous to Eysenck, Raymond Cattell (1905–1998) also used statistical analysis to identify 16 personality factors. These 16 personality factors were then categorized into five "global" or second-order factors: Extraversion, Anxiety, Tough-Mindedness, Independence, and Self-Control. The first two factors, Extraversion and Anxiety, are conceptually similar to Eysenck's dimensions of Extraversion and Neuroticism. Tough-mindedness relates to a person's openness (or lack thereof) to new ideas; the opposite of "tough-mindedness" is "receptivity." Independence is related to the tendency to be self-determining or dominant versus deferential; the opposite of "independence" is "accommodation." Finally, self-control can be correlated with Eysenck's dimension of Psychoticism. In the Cattell model, the opposite of "self-control" is "lack of restraint." Like Eysenck, Cattell believed that biology, and in particular genetics, are the basis of the personality factors, and therefore, the factors are stable over time and experience.

TABLE 8–1. Cattell's 16 Personality Factors and Five Global Factors

Dimensions of Personality	
Factor A	Warmth (Reserved vs. Warm)
Factor B	Reasoning (Concrete vs. Abstract)
Factor C	Emotional Stability (Reactive vs. Emotionally Stable)
Factor E	Dominance (Deferential vs. Dominant)
Factor F	Liveliness (Serious vs. Lively)
Factor G	Rule-Consciousness (Expedient vs. Rule-Conscious)
Factor H	Social Boldness (Shy vs. Socially Bold)
Factor I	Sensitivity (Utilitarian vs. Sensitive)
Factor L	Vigilance (Trusting vs. Vigilant)
Factor M	Abstractedness (Grounded vs. Abstracted)
Factor N	Privateness (Forthright vs. Private)
Factor O	Apprehension (Self-Assured vs. Apprehensive)
Factor Q1	Openness to Change (Traditional vs. Open to Change)
Factor Q2	Self-Reliance (Group-Oriented vs. Self-Reliant)
Factor Q3	Perfectionism (Tolerates Disorder vs. Perfectionistic)
Factor Q4	Tension (Relaxed vs. Tense)
Global Factors	
EX	Extraversion
ANX	Anxiety
TM	Tough-Mindedness
IN	Independence
SC	Self-Control

The traits-based models of personality were dominant throughout the 1950's and 60's, until a schism was opened in personality psychology by Walter Mischel (1930–) with the publication of his book *Personality and Assessment* in 1968. Mischel (1973) argued that a critical flaw of the "global dispositional approaches" (i.e., the traits-based models of personality) was the failure to consider physical and social environments. For example, teenagers might behave differently around their friends than around parents or teachers. And baseball players might behave differently in a preseason exhibition game than in a deciding seventh game in the World Series. Mischel (1973) promoted a theory of personality that incorporated concepts of social learning theory. Debate was vigorous. Reviews of Mischel's 1968 book were not all favorable, and Eysenck and his son (also a psychologist) published a dismissive rebuttal to Mischel's ideas in 1980. Decades of argument did result in some compromise, and today, most personality theorists acknowledge that there are both stable elements of personality (traits) and an influence of the environment.

Today, the prevailing model of personality is known as the "Big Five" and it resembles the five global personality traits identified by Cattell in the 1950's. This model was developed and advocated by Goldberg (1990) and a questionnaire to assess the five global traits (named similarly, but not identically) was published by Costa and McCrae in 1992. The current version of the Costa and McCrae questionnaire is called the NEO-PI-3, where "PI" stands for personality inventory and "NEO" originally referenced neuroticism, extraversion, and openness (the original questionnaire assessed only these three factors, two more were later added). More commonly, the NEO-PI-3 is known by the acronym OCEAN, from the first letter of each of the five factors.

TABLE 8–2. Measurements of the NEO-PI-3

- **Neuroticism** (Anxiety, Hostility, Depression, Self-Consciousness, Impulsiveness, Vulnerability)
- **Extraversion** (Warmth, Gregariousness, Assertiveness, Activity, Excitement-Seeking, Positive Emotions)
- **Openness to Experience** (Fantasy, Aesthetics, Feelings, Actions, Ideas, Values)
- **Agreeableness** (Trust, Modesty, Compliance, Altruism, Straightforwardness, Tender-Mindedness)
- **Conscientiousness** (Competence, Self-Discipline, Achievement-Striving, Dutifulness, Order, Deliberation)

From: http://www.sigmaassessmentsystems.com/assessments/neopi3.asp

---

Assignment 8–2.   Try to map the words and phrases you used to describe your own personality to the Big Five factors (see Table 8–2). Do you have a word or phrase for each of the five factors? Do you think you would score high or low for each of the five?

Personality research applied to athletics has generally found that competitive sports participants score higher for extraversion and lower for neuroticism than non-athletes (Eagleton et. al., 2007; McKelvie et. al., 2003; Tripathi, 1980). When the Big Five inventory was applied to fitness center members, the results were similar; members were more likely to score high for extraversion and low for neuroticism (Chen et. al., 2007). A natural question is to ask is whether the 'athletic' personality type is a cause or an effect. Do more extraverted, less anxious people choose to play competitive sports (the gravitational hypothesis) or does playing competitive sports tend to make a person more extraverted and less anxious? A study of college sports athletes demonstrated no change in the Eysenck Personality Inventory over the four years of participation, suggesting that more extraverted personalities are attracted to sports participation, rather than that sports participation affected personality (Eagleton et. al., 2007).

Assignment 8–3.   Prior studies have indicated that in general, competitive athletes score higher for extraversion and lower for neuroticism than non-athletes. (a) Do you think there is a difference between team and non-team athletes (e.g., basketball players versus tennis players)? If yes, on which of the Big Five parameters? (b) How do you think competitive card players or chess players might score on the Big Five parameters? Do you think they would be similar to athletes or different? Why? Can you find any scientific studies to support (or refute) your guesses?

Aggression

We all know individuals whom we would describe (in terms of their personality) as "aggressive". What do we mean by that? From a theoretical stand point, the answer is not simple. For example, in his book *Rethinking Aggression and Violence in Sport*, author John Kerr devotes six pages to the definition of "aggressive." The American Psychological Association defines aggression as "behaviors that cause psychological or physical harm to another individual." However, athletes, coaches and fans all recognize in sports "aggressive" behavior that does not fit this definition. For example, if a track athlete aggressively pushes to the front of a pack, that individual is jockeying for position, not attempting to hurt someone else. For our context, we will describe that type of behavior—behavior intended to gain a tactical advantage but not injure, as "assertive" (Husman and Silva, 1984 in Kerr, 2005). Nonetheless, examples of aggressive behavior, as the American Psychological Society defines it, abound in sport, involving not only athletes, but also coaches and fans.

Researchers have categorized aggressive behaviors according to the motivation or intent of the aggressor. Hostile aggression is motivated by the intent to injure another while instrumental aggression is behavior that does injure, but is motivated by another goal (e.g., to score or gain a tactical advantage). Kerr (2005) distinguished four types of aggression in sports, again separated according to the aggressor's motivation—play, anger, power, and thrill (Table 8–3). An example of instrumental, play aggression occurs when a football player injures another during a legal tackle. National Hockey League (NHL) hockey games annually provide many examples of hostile aggression, including anger, power, and thrill aggression. Before we continue to a case example from the NHL, we will discuss hypotheses that have been proposed to explain aggressive behavior.

TABLE 8–3. Types of Aggressive Behavior in Sports According to Kerr (2005)

Type of Aggressive Behavior	Permitted or Not Permitted in Sport?	Hostile or Instrumental?	Description
Play	Yes	Instrumental	Assertive behavior—legal or sanctioned within the sport
Anger	No	Hostile	Provoked by recent event, often retaliatory
Power	No	Hostile	Intending to intimidate
Thrill	No	Hostile	Intended to provoke

Aggressive behavior is not limited to humans. For example, when two male deer spar over does, or two fish fight over territory, they are exhibiting aggression. We attribute the innate aggressive behavior of animals to their genetics and physiology. Research focused on animals led to the development of deterministic (biological) theories to explain human aggressive behavior (Kerr, 2005). These theories are not well supported. In 1939, the frustration-aggression hypothesis was proposed by Dollard and several colleagues at Yale University (Eron, 1994). According to this proposal, individuals build up frustration as they are thwarted in various ways, and that frustration inevitably leads to an aggressive act. This theory also proved inadequate to explain the range of human aggressive behavior (as well as the range in response to frustration) (Eron, 1994). Social learning theory provides an alternate explanation for aggressive behavior.

According to social learning theory, aggressive behavior is learned from influential others such as parents, teachers, coaches, and peers (Eron, 1994). Aggressive behavior occurs when the *expected reward outweighs the expected punishment*. The aggressor's expectations for reward and punishment are informed by the explicit and tacit rules of the event, as well as by learned social cues. Aggressive acts are encouraged by a permissive atmosphere. If officials overlook rather than penalize a hostile aggressive act (for example, intentionally stepping on or kicking an opponent who is on the ground), then that action, while not technically legal by the rules of the game (most likely), is, in fact, permitted. The risk of punishment is low. Socialization to sanctioned deviance is another environmental condition that can promote aggressive behavior. Sanctioned deviance refers to behaviors that are technically illegal but in practice accepted by society. Examples of sanctioned deviance include driving a car at 60 miles per hour when the speed limit is 55 miles per hour. If I asked you, "Why did you drive 60 miles per hour when you know the speed limit is only 55?" you might answer "It's okay because everybody does it." You know that the risk of punishment (i.e., a speeding ticket) is low. Fist fighting is often permitted and sanctioned in hockey, even in youth hockey. In fact, youth hockey fighting camps have been offered to teach young players how to be "goons" (Blount, 2007). The potential rewards for aggressive behavior include praise, status, and tactical advantage. Praise may come from a coach, other players, and spectators. Likewise, elevated status can be conferred by teammates or others. A recent study found that when heterosexual women were shown photographs of men who were described as non-athletes, casual athletes, competitive but non-aggressive athletes, or competitive, aggressive athletes, the women rated the men identified as competitive, aggressive athletes as the most desirable for a short or long-term relationship (Brewer and Howarth, 2012). This study reflects our social environment, and according to social learning theory, societal cues affect behavior.

A Case Study in Sports Aggression or Violence

In a February, 2004 NHL game, Steve Moore of the Colorado Avalanche injured Markus Naslund of the Vancouver Canucks. The play was deemed legal and no penalty was assessed, although Naslund suffered a concussion and missed three games. The Canucks were outraged and one of their players declared that there was a "bounty" on Steve Moore. In a game in March 2004, the Canucks "enforcer," Todd Bertuzzi, a player whose unofficial job included retaliatory (anger) aggression, attempted to taunt Moore into a fight. Failing at that, he intentionally hit Moore from behind. Moore fell to the ice face first, unconscious, with Bertuzzi falling on him. Moore left the ice on a stretcher and was subsequently diagnosed with three fractured cervical vertebrae and a concussion. Bertuzzi was ejected from the game, suspended for the remainder of the season, and fined $500,000 by the NHL. The NHL also fined the Canucks operation $250,000 for what they called a "conducive atmosphere." The Canucks were shocked to be implicated. In criminal court, Bertuzzi was charged with assault and accepted a plea bargain of one year of probation, a small fine, and community service. The NHL reinstated Bertuzzi for the 2005–2006 season, and he continued to play through the 2012–2013 season. Steve Moore had permanent injuries and did not play again. In 2006, Moore filed a civil lawsuit against Bertuzzi and the Canucks for $38 million dollars of lost income and punitive damages. The trial has been delayed several times and remains unsettled. The disclosure that the New Orleans Saints football team offered a "bounty" for its players who seriously injured an opposing player prompted Lester Munson of ESPN.com to write a commentary on the Bertuzzi-Moore incident and its implications for the NFL and other sports organizations. The commentary link is below.

http://espn.go.com/espn/commentary/story/_/page/munson-120315/todd-bertuzzi-hit-steve -moore-2004-cautionary-tale-new-orleans-saints-bounties

As noted above, fighting is permitted and sanctioned in hockey. Kerr (2006) has summarized, "Although it is considered an act of unsanctioned violence in sports like rugby, American football, and Australian rules football . . . fist-fighting still retains a special status within North American, and especially NHL, ice hockey. Indeed, it could be said to be sanctioned, as it is freely engaged in by many players, used as a tactic by coaches, expected by fans, and tolerated by officials and administrators."

Assignment 8–4. Who or what is to blame for Steve Moore's career-ending injuries? Do you blame Todd Bertuzzi, Bertuzzi's coach or team, the NHL officials, the NHL itself, or all of these parties? Can the permissive atmosphere for hostile aggression in NHL hockey be changed? How would that change be achieved? Are problems with hostile aggression in sports limited to players or do you think that problems also exist in the realm of sports fans?

Interestingly, both instrumental and hostile aggression do not appear to differ by gender, at least in adult competitive sports. Keeler (2007) looked at male and female collision sport (rugby), contact sport (soccer) and non-contact sport (volleyball) players' aggressive behaviors. When controlling for age, experience, and level of success, the study found equal degrees of both instrumental and hostile aggression in men and women. The study also found no differences between athletes in the sports of different contact levels, contrary to findings in youth athletics.

Motivation

Motivation encompasses a person's choice of goals, as well as intensity and persistence of goal pursuit. For example, can we predict which individuals will choose to pursue physical fitness? Can we predict which individuals will work hard toward this goal, and not give up? Research in motivation seeks to address these types of questions.

Psychologists differentiate between intrinsic and extrinsic motivation. Intrinsic motivation comes from within, and is based on natural enjoyment of a particular activity. In sports, we might describe intrinsic motivation as "love of the game." Extrinsic motivation is based on external rewards—money, fame, trophies, etc. Generally, feedback that reinforces a person's sense of competency will increase intrinsic motivation (Ryan and Deci, 2000). Praise, a sense of self-control, and success are examples of external information that strengthen self-confidence and intrinsic motivation. In contrast, external rewards tend to undermine intrinsic motivation (Deci et al., 1999). For example, consider a person who chooses to convert a hobby such as painting or writing into his nine to five job. In that case, what was a recreational activity becomes work—and it may seem less enjoyable.

The theory of achievement motivation, which was developed in the late 1950's, posits that motivation is the combined effect of three factors: a trait variable called motive, which is a person's inherent need for achievement; a task characteristic called expectancy, which is the perceived probability of success; and the value of the task, which is measured by the pride and self-satisfaction that accrue from success (Weiner, 2010). Expectancy and value are inversely related because tasks that are perceived as easy (very high probability of success) provide low value (pride upon success), whereas tasks that are perceived to be very hard will yield high value if the performer is successful. The trait variable motive is a personality construct. Individuals can be rated along a continuum from low to high motive. Some individuals have high achievement motivation, and strive for success and internal reward, whereas others have lower achievement motivation. The achievement motivation theory predicts that individuals with high motive will tend to select tasks of intermediate difficulty because those tasks have the highest combination of expectancy (chance of success) and value. Bernard Weiner, a student of achievement motivation theory in the early 1960's, recognized some of the theory's shortfalls, and with collaborators, built upon it and developed attribution theory.

Attribution theory focuses on the attributions, or reasons, that individuals give for their successes and failures. For example, students may explain high or low class grades, and athletes may explain wins and losses. According to attribution theory, there are four fundamental attributions: ability, effort, task difficulty, and luck. Attributions can be *internal* to the person (ability, effort) or *external* (task difficulty, luck). Attributions can also be either *stable* (ability, task difficulty) or *unstable* and rapidly changeable (effort, luck). Attribution theory ties a person's attributions about a success or failure to future task selection, investment, and perseverance. In other words, attributions affect motivation and allow us to predict behavior. Imagine a student who fails calculus. If she attributes her failure to missing classes and neglecting homework, in essence, to a lack of effort, then her hope for future success may be maintained and she may choose to re-take the class. If, on the other hand, she attributes her failure to a lack of math aptitude, then hope for future success is not bright and she may change majors or even leave school.

In general, people make attributions that protect their ego by promoting a sense of self-efficacy, or task specific self-confidence. To bolster self-efficacy, individuals tend to attribute successes to internal factors and failures to external factures. For example, an investor who attributes financial gain to hard work is making an internal attribution, while an investor who attributes financial losses to bad luck in market timing is making an external attribution. These are known as self-serving attributions. The more an individual is personally invested in, or cares about, an outcome, the more likely he or she will invoke a self-serving attribution. Consequently, if you do not think of yourself as a good singer, and singing is not part of your identity, you may be willing to say that a loss in a singing contest is due to poor ability. If you were a vocal performance major, you would not be likely to make the same attribution. Studies have shown that attribution of failure to effort, which is both controllable and changeable, promotes more task perseverance than attributions of failure to a stable cause such as task difficulty (e.g., LeFoll et. al., 2008).

Assignment 8–5.   Find an example of an athlete making a causal attribution for a sports success/win or failure/loss in a print or on-line article. Which of the four fundamental attributions best describes the athlete's declared reason for the competition outcome? Is the attribution self-serving?

The attributions a person gives for a success or failure can depend on who will witness the attribution. If a tennis player is asked by a reporter why he lost a match, he can more easily blame bad referee calls or poor environmental conditions (i.e., luck) than he can if he is asked by a fellow tennis player who is a better judge of tennis ability—of the player and his opponent. Attributions made by team members for team play tend to be less biased then are attributions made by individuals for their own performance. However, the more closely allied individual ego is with team performance, the more self-serving team attributions become.

Assignment 8–6. If you were the coach of a National Basketball Association (NBA) team, would you want to attribute a team loss to players of low ability or to being "outplayed"? What are the implications of each potential attribution? What is the likely effect of each potential attribution on subsequent player practice ethic?

Group Dynamics

In comparing individual and team attributions, we are touching on an area of study called group dynamics. Group dynamics are important to any team, whether that be an athletic team, a sales team, a fire-fighting team, a construction team, etc. That said, team members are not the only individuals a performer may interact with; there may also be others performing the same activity either in competition or not in direct competition, and there may be spectators. When you take a final exam in a room full of classmates who are also taking a final exam, you are in a room of co-actors—individuals performing the same activity you are performing. Those individuals are not in direct competition with you, unlike, for example, runners in a race. If you act in a play in front of an audience, in addition to your co-actors on stage, you are performing in front of an auditorium full of observers. Group dynamics addresses the influence of competitors, co-actors, and observers on behavior, particularly, performance. Think back to the study by Triplett that was described at the beginning of this chapter. What did Triplett conclude was the impact of competitors on the cyclists' performance?

Classic studies by Robert Zajonc (pronounced "zions") led to the conclusion that, in general, observers or co-actors facilitate (improve) the performance of easy and familiar tasks but impair the performance of difficult or novel tasks (Zajonc, 1965). Characteristics of the observers can impact behavior. For example, aggressive behavior is promoted if subjects believe their audience is a boxing club, whereas aggressive behavior is decreased if subjects believe their audience is a pacifist club. Consider your own behavior in class, in front of classmates and teachers, in comparison to your behavior in an informal setting, in front of only your friends. Are there differences? Are you more talkative or forthcoming with your opinions in one setting than in the other? Are you more likely to utter swear words in one setting than in the other?

Team "chemistry" is a feature that coaches often cite as important to team success. What coaches call "chemistry", a psychologist would call "cohesion." Cohesion is the tendency of group members to remain united in pursuit of a goal (wins, sales, putting out fires, construction, etc.). Coaches are correct that high team cohesion promotes attainment of team goals, however the causality is circular—team success also promotes group cohesion. When a team is winning, members tend to get along well and remain united. Cohesion may crumble when a team faces adversity. Good coaches and managers employ techniques known to promote team cohesion. Those techniques include small group size, physical proximity, excellent communication, role differentiation, conformity, and low permeability. If a team is large, such as a 90 to 100 member college football roster, then to promote cohesion, the team can be broken down into subgroups, for example, receivers, linebackers, offensive linemen, etc. The same is true in business, in which the employees may be put into departments such as a development, customer support, and marketing (etc.). Physical proximity, as long as it is not excessive, promotes communication and cohesion. Managers must recognize an appropriate level of physical proximity. Many professional teams run a pre-season camp in which players eat, sleep and practice together, but those camps are of limited duration. Communication, both task-oriented and social, promotes cohesion. Hence, meetings about goals and strategy are important, as are informal "water cooler" conversations. Role differentiation means that each individual member should have a distinct job, but furthermore, that individual must understand and accept his or her role. For example, if a player is a relief pitcher, that player must understand and accept that he will not play until the lead pitcher comes out of the game. Although role differentiation has a positive impact on cohesion, conformity in other respects also promotes cohesion. Matching clothing in the sense of a uniform or dress code is perhaps the most ubiquitous way to promote cohesion through conformity. Permeability, the degree to which team members communicate with individuals outside the team, detracts from cohesion. No coach or business manager encourages team members to communicate with the competition!

Arousal

In the psychological context, arousal refers to the continuum of awareness states between sleep (very low arousal) and hypervigilant (very high arousal). Obviously, very low levels of arousal are not ideal for performance of most tasks. You would not want to be asleep during your final exam and you would not wish your team's goalie to be nodding off in the net. At the same time, extremely high levels of arousal are not ideal for many tasks, either. Very high arousal levels can be perceived as anxiety or "stress."

The inverted U hypothesis summarizes these observations. This theory describes the effect of arousal on performance quality. For any given activity, there exists an optimal arousal level.

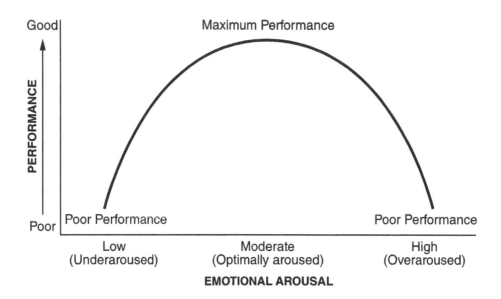

FIGURE 8-3. The inverted U hypothesis. Performance improves with arousal level up to an optimal arousal point. As arousal increases further, performance quality declines. Williams et. al., 1993.

Williams et. al., 1993.

Both individuals and coaches have a sense of the optimal arousal level for different tasks. For example, what type of music do athletes choose before competitions? Do you think precision athletes like archers would choose to listen to the same type of music before competition as power athletes like football players or shot put throwers? Fans and coaches also help to modulate player arousal levels. Fans will cheer loudly and wildly at times, but typically, the home crowd will be relatively quiet when its team is at (for example) the free throw line. Coaches have to know when to rile up a player, and when to put a player on the bench to cool off.

Assignment 8–7.   Draw a graph to illustrate the relationship between arousal and performance in golf driving (a power activity) and golf putting (a precision activity). Use the same axes as shown in Figure 8–3.

Arousal relates to the relative simulation of the sympathetic versus parasympathetic systems. When the sympathetic nervous system is activated, epinephrine (adrenaline) is released from the adrenal glands. Caffeine, which antagonizes or blocks adenosine receptors in the brain, also increases arousal. In contrast, alcohol decreases arousal. General arousal theory postulates that arousal itself is physiological, but the conscious perception of physiological state is informed by the environment. A clever test of general arousal theory was published by Dutton and Aron in 1974. They used a female confederate (an undercover researcher) to stop and question men as the men crossed two very different bridges. One bridge, the Capilano bridge in British Columbia, Canada is one of the world's highest and longest suspension bridges. It sways when it is traversed and most people find the experience scary, i.e., arousing. In contrast, the other bridge was low and solid, in short, not scary at all. One of the outcome variables was how many of the men interviewed on each of the bridges accepted the confederate's phone number and chose to call her later. More men interviewed on the scary bridge than on the unthreatening bridge did so. The interpretation of this finding was that the experience of crossing the Capilano bridge created a physiological state of arousal that the men interpreted as sexual attraction. The romance between the two lead characters of the 1994 movie *Speed*, starring Sandra Bullock and Keanu Reeves, is based on the same premise. The two characters go through a terrifying experience together, and fall in love.

References

Blount, R. 2007. "Last Thing Hockey Needs is a Fighting Camp for Kids." Minneapolis *Star Tribune*. July 16.

Brewer, G. and Howarth, S. 2012. "Sport, Attractiveness, and Aggression." *Personality and Individual Differences*. Netherlands: Elsevier.

Deci, E., Koestner, R., and Ryan R. M. 1999. "A Meta-analytic Review of Experiments Examining the Effects of Extrinsic Rewards on Intrinsic Motivation." *Psychological Bulletin* 125(6):627–68.

Eysenck, H. 1947. *Dimensions of Personality*. epublished by the Library of Congress 1997.

Eysenck, M. and Eysenck, H. Mischel and the concept of personality. *British J. Psychology*. 71(2):191–205, 1980.

Green, C.D. Psychology strikes out: Coleman R. Griffith and the Chicago Cubs. *Hist. Psychol.* 6(3):267–283, 2003.

Howarth, E. What does Eysenck's psychoticism scale really measure? *Br. J. Psychol.* 77(2):223–7, 1986.

Keeler, L. A. The differences in sport aggression, life aggression, and life assertion among adult male and female collision, contact, and non-contact sport athletes. *Journal of Sport Behavior.* 30(1):57–76, 2007.

Kerr, J. H. 2005. *Rethinking Aggression and Violence in Sports.* New York: Taylor & Francis.

Kremer, J. and Moran, A. 2008. "Swifter, Higher, Stronger: The History of Sport Psychology." *The Psychologist* 21(8):740–2.

Lykken, D. 2011. Lykken on Leadership. Communication and Leadership (Part 1). *National Mortgage Professional Magazine,* November. Retrieved from http://nationalmortgageprofessional.com/news27361/lykken-leadership -communication-and-leadership-part-1.

March, A. W. 1952. "The Educational Values of College Physical Education, Including Intercollegiate Athletics, and Their Preservation." *The Educational Forum* 16(4):409–19.

Triplett, N. 1898. "The Dynamogenic Factors in Pacemaking and Competition." *American Journal of Psychology* 9:507–33.

Weiner, B. 2010. "The Development of an Attribution-based Theory of Motivation: A History of Ideas." *Educational Psychologist* 45(1):28–36.

Chapter 9

WHAT CAN YOU DO WITH A DEGREE IN EXERCISE SCIENCE?

As you know from Chapter 1, the field of Exercise Science has changed a great deal in the last quarter century, going from individual courses studied by Health and Physical Education students, to a field unto itself. With that change has come a dramatic expansion in the career fields pursued by Exercise Science majors. This chapter will provide a brief overview of careers that are available to you as you graduate in exercise science.

Exercise Science graduates may choose from a wide array of graduate school opportunities. Many students major in exercise science with the goal of entering a graduate program in the health professions. Examples of these include Physical and Occupational Therapy, Physician Assistant, and Medicine. Exercise Science is an excellent major for students desiring entry into these schools since it is often one of the few majors in a university that has as its emphasis the anatomy and physiology of humans, which is a great advantage for these career paths. There are many other career paths students can take into the workplace following a degree in Exercise Science, some of which can be quite lucrative.

Careers Directly Following a Bachelor's Degree in Exercise Science

Many students plan to seek a job immediately following an undergraduate degree. In some cases, this plan follows a specific career choice; in others, it may be to pay down undergraduate student debt prior to moving on to graduate school, or to gain experience to better determine whether graduate and professional training are what the student wants. Regardless of the reason, there are numerous choices of careers that a person may pursue with an undergraduate Exercise Science degree. This section will give an overview of some of them.

Cardiac and Pulmonary Rehabilitation/Clinical Exercise Physiologist

Historically, cardiopulmonary rehabilitation has been a major source of employment for students with an undergraduate degree in Exercise Science. In fact, some baccalaureate programs emphasize this training for their students. Many clinical exercise physiologists work in cardiac rehabilitation settings, while others work in facilities such as hospitals, universities, and stress testing centers. Clinical exercise physiologists administer exercise tests, generally under the supervision of a physician, develop and monitor exercise programs, and coordinate the range of education needed by patients who have suffered a cardiovascular or pulmonary event (e.g., a "heart attack") requiring rehabilitation. Patient education usually includes the benefits and risks of exercise and how to incorporate exercise into a lifestyle. It often also includes diet and nutrition education in conjunction with a dietician, as well as education on diseases that patients may also have including diabetes, cardiovascular or pulmonary disease, or other diseases that affect exercise capability and can often be improved by exercise.

There is a widely recognized certification for clinical exercise physiologists, the Registered Clinical Exercise Physiologist or RCEP®. The RCEP is offered by the American College of Sports Medicine (ACSM), and requires specialized training, career experience and a certification examination. Most clinical exercise physiologists, though, begin their careers without this certification and gain on-the-job experience while working toward certification. The ACSM also offers an Exercise Specialist® certification that requires only 500 hours of clinical exercise physiology experience and passing a certification exam. Entry-level exercise physiologist positions generally require a bachelor's degree in Exercise Science, Kinesiology, or a related field. Students interested in entering the field of clinical exercise physiology should also have one or more internships as part of their undergraduate career to gain experience prior to graduating. In some fortunate cases, an internship may transform into a job.

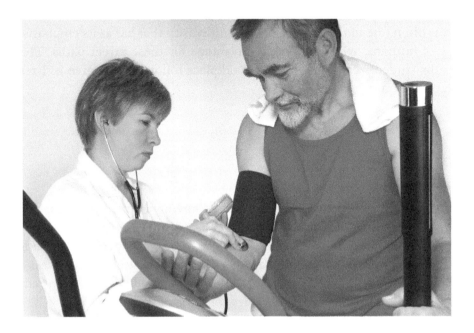

FIGURE 9–1. Cardiac rehabilitation practitioner with patient.

© Alexander Raths, 2013. Used under license from Shutterstock, Inc.

Salaries in cardiac rehabilitation vary widely depending on the level of experience, as well as the area of the country in which the clinical exercise physiologist is employed. Typical starting salaries in 2010–2012 were $25,000–$35,000 with the median salary in the United States averaging $45,000–$52,000 (cardiacrehabilitationsalary.com, simplyhired.com, cepa-acsm.org). There are two national organizations that specialize in clinical exercise physiology and cardiac and pulmonary rehabilitation. These are the Clinical Exercise Physiology Association (CEPA), which is an affiliate of the American College of Sports Medicine (www.cepa-acsm.org) and the American Association for Cardiovascular and Pulmonary Rehabilitation (AACVPR) (www.aacvpr.org). The websites for these organizations are excellent starting points to learn more about the field and what is required to enter into them.

Personal Training

Personal training is a rapidly growing area that involves a fitness specialist working one-on-one or with a group of clients to improve their health and fitness. The training may be done in a gym or recreation facility, or in the privacy of the client's home. Different from cardiac or pulmonary rehabilitation, personal trainers work with apparently healthy populations, not people with known cardiovascular or other diseases that could make exercise harmful for them. Several organizations offer certifications in personal training including the ACSM (certification.acsm.org /acsm-certified-personal-trainer) and the American Council on Exercise (http://www.acefitness .org/fitness-certifications/personal-trainer-certification/default.aspx). In most cases the minimum qualifications do not require a college degree, although a good working knowledge of the human body and how it responds to exercise would be very valuable, for obvious reasons. Some exercise science students gain real-world experience and maybe a career by starting as personal trainers while they are still working on their degrees.

Salaries for personal trainers vary widely. Beginning trainers often make $12–$15 per hour, with average wages up to $35,000 to $50,000 per year (www.nfpt.com; www.indeed.com). The range of salaries is based on experience, the locale in which the trainer works, and what the trainer offers the client.

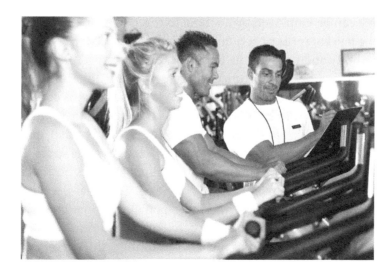

FIGURE 9–2. Personal trainer working with several clients.

Corporate Fitness/Wellness

The field of corporate fitness incorporates a number of different areas of study, one of which is exercise science. A corporate fitness specialist is usually a company employee, but may be a consultant to many corporations. The primary goal of a corporate fitness program is to increase productivity in the workplace, both by making more attentive and fit employees and by decreasing medical costs (Blaiker, et al., 2010), thus lowering both sick time and insurance costs for the company.

A corporate fitness specialist will help companies organize fitness programs, dietary counseling, smoking cessation and many other health-related activities. The fitness portion may include something as simple as adding a small fitness center in a company's location or providing gym memberships for its employees. It may, though, include a large corporate fitness facility with a range of exercise machines, classes, and one-on-one fitness counseling, for which a well-trained fitness specialist might be required. The fitness specialist would not only monitor exercise programs, but would also be responsible for increasing the participation of employees, for making sure the exercise environment is safe and welcoming to employees, and for providing the corporate executives evidence of the effectiveness of the program. Therefore, many corporate fitness specialists will have some training in exercise techniques and motivating people, but will also likely have enough background in the business of exercise to be able to document the effectiveness of the program. Some of this experience will be gained in the classroom, but some will come about as a result of internships and on-the-job training. Median salaries for those employed as corporate fitness specialists for major companies in 2010 was between $67,000 and $79,000 (www.indeed.com; www.simplyhired.com).

Coaching

A very broad field, coaching entails teaching athletes at different levels, the basic and advanced techniques involved in a sport or strength conditioning. Coaching ranges from working with students at the pre- and grammar school level to instructing professional athletes on the nuances of batting or a golf swing. Many, but not all, coaches at the K-12 level also have teaching certificates so that they can be employed by a school to teach in a content area in addition to their sport. Regardless of the level of sport or activity at which a person coaches, a good degree of familiarity with the human body and its anatomy and physiology, is a useful part of the training. Current and accurate knowledge of human function helps prevent unnecessary injuries and illness sometimes associated with simply coaching the way a person's previous coach did.

In addition, it is obvious that to be an effective coach, an intimate knowledge of the sport or activity is necessary. This knowledge often comes from personally participating in the activity, and it is not uncommon for a star athlete to become a coach in her/his sport. Personal experience in the sport is not absolutely necessary, though, as there are examples both of people who participated, but did not excel at the national or international level, as well as people who got into coaching after having been team managers, without ever playing a sport competitively. Regardless, coaching is a time-absorbing career that encompasses many activities beyond working with an athlete on sport skills. These other activities include recruiting, athlete counseling and regulatory compliance, scheduling and dealing with parents and fans among other things, and a person must expect to work his/her way "up the ranks" to gain much monetary advantage from the profession. Incoming coaches may work for no compensation (as volunteers) and often enter the profession as graduate assistants. While head coaches in marquee sports can make millions of dollars a year, most make a fraction of that amount.

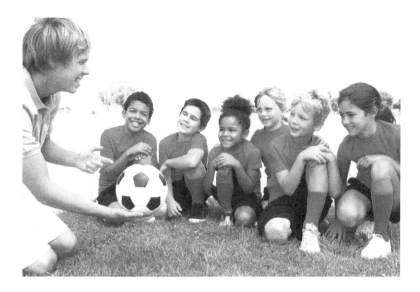

FIGURE 9–3. Coach working with youth soccer players.
© Monkey Business Images, 2013. Used under license from Shutterstock, Inc.

Pharmaceutical and Medical Implement Sales

Although pharmaceutical and medical implement sales is not a field discussed much among Exercise Science majors, it is a viable option for someone who desires to enter the job market upon graduation. Since Exercise Science is one of the few majors offered at many universities that focuses on human studies in the physiological realm, it can be good good preparation for entry into the medical sales field. Pharmaceutical and medical implement sales involves contact with individual physicians and other health care providers, as well as with hospitals and insurance companies. The salesperson's goal is to have their product directly purchased by the client, or included among the products sold or supported by the client. This position also involves a great deal of on-the-job education. The sales representative is expected to know each of his/her products in great detail, from mechanism of action to indications and contraindications for its use. The position often involves a great deal of travel, depending on the territory in which the representative works (Princeton Review, online). The sales representative position by itself does not provide a large amount of upward mobility, but it does provide avenues into the corporation that would not generally be available for someone outside the company. Sales representatives in this area can expect to earn up to $73,000 as a median, with larger salaries for productive representatives with ideal product lines (www.salary.com).

Careers that Require Education Beyond a Bachelor's Degree

Most Exercise Science majors in recent years have a career goal that requires education beyond, and in some cases much beyond, a bachelor's degree. Many Exercise Science majors progress to professional training to obtain a career in a clinical field. This type of education can take as little as two years (post bachelor's degree), or as much as ten or more years, depending on the field and on the specialty within that field.

Physical Therapy

A physical therapist works with individual patients to increase strength, function, and mobility. They also work with clients to help prevent loss of these attributes due to aging or disease processes. A physical therapist may work with patients from neonates to centenarians in a variety of settings including clinics, hospitals, homes, schools, and performance facilities.

An undergraduate degree in Exercise Science is commonly considered a very good preparation for physical therapy (PT) training, since it involves a large number of science courses and concentrates on human movement, but it is not required—any undergraduate degree may be acceptable as long as the PT program entry requirements are met. While most PT programs require a bachelor's degree for entry, there are a few "3+3" programs in the country, where a student can gain entry into PT school after their third year of college and complete the PT degree in an additional three years. Virtually all PT programs in the US now offer the doctor of physical therapy (DPT) degree, and all will be *required* to do by 2015 (APTA). While specific entry requirements vary by program, most PT programs require General Biology, Chemistry and Physics, as well Human Anatomy and Physiology, Statistics, and Psychology. In addition, clinical experience prior to admission, or even before an interview, is considered important. Some programs have specific requirements for the amount and type of clinical experience, while others do not. Regardless of the requirements, it is useful to have as much and as varied experience in patient care, broadly, and in physical therapy, specifically, as possible. This experience will help the student be sure that PT is the right field of choice based on knowledge and not simply because it sounds exciting. Students interested in PT school should begin looking into programs and requirements early in their undergraduate program. Doing so will help the student make sure of having all the requirements, both academic and clinical, prior to beginning the application process. The application process for most PT programs is now on-line through the Physical Therapy Central Application Service (PTCAS). Students would be wise to become familiar with this service prior to beginning the application process.

Once in PT school, what should a student expect? PT school courses include ones that one would expect, such as courses in muscle and neural biology, pharmacology, physiology and biomechanics. The PT student should also expect to take courses in psychology and sociology, as well as the business of physical therapy. Courses typically comprise approximately 80% of the curriculum, with clinical experience taking the remaining 20% (APTA). Once this training is completed, the student must pass a licensing examination in the state in which he or she wants to practice.

With the aging of the population, PTs, like most other health professionals, are expected to be in increased demand. Physical therapist salaries, like those of most other professions, vary with the practice, setting and area of the country where the PT practices. Salaries for PTs start around $50,000 and the median salary is approximately $76,000 (medical-careers-review; Bureau of Labor Statistics). The primary professional organization for PTs is the American Physical Therapy Association (APTA), and it would be valuable for any student desiring to become a PT to become familiar with the association.

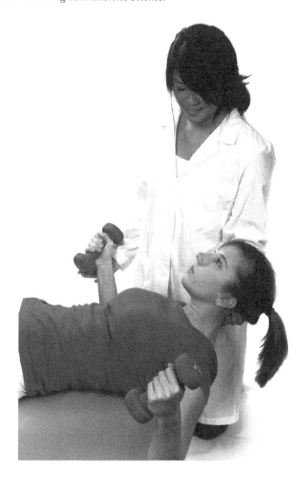

FIGURE 9-4. Physical therapist with a patient.
© aceshot, 2013. Used under license from Shutterstock, Inc.

Occupational Therapy

An occupational therapist (OT) works with patients to maintain or regain skills needed for acts of daily living. Some of the techniques used are similar to those involved in PT while others are not, and often OTs and PTs work together with patients to help them regain their function following an accident, stroke or other incident. While a bit oversimplified, a basic rule of thumb is that PTs work to help patients move freely and perform large muscle activities, while OTs work to help patients with fine motor skills like dressing, eating, and brushing teeth (for examples). An OT will typically evaluate a patient, and then assist the person with both activities to help them improve their skills and with changes to the living environment to help the patient be able to perform necessary activities with the diminished skills that may be present. The work of an OT may be in a clinic, hospital, school or patient's home.

The entry requirements for most OT programs include a bachelor's degree, but the undergraduate major is not specified. Typical majors include biology, exercise science and psychology, but like most other health professions, the major is not the important thing, rather it is most important to have the courses required for admission. Therefore, it is critical to contact programs in which you might be interested in order to make sure you have the required courses for entry.

Once in OT school, courses in physiology and anatomy, therapeutic modalities, and managing a practice will be common. Fieldwork as well as class work are key elements of OT education. Following completion of the degree you will have to take a national certification examination in order to practice.

Occupational therapists' job outlook is very bright with the population demographics as they are, and the salaries are competitive with many other health professions. Median salaries are currently approximately $73,000, with entry salaries of approximately $50,000 (Bureau of Labor Statistics; money.usnews.com). The professional organization for occupational therapists is the American Occupational Therapy Association (AOTA). Students interested in this field should make themselves familiar with this organization.

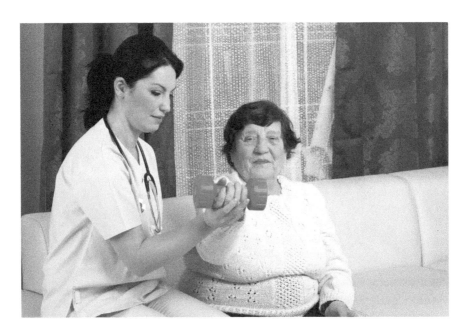

FIGURE 9–5: Occupational therapist with patient.

Blaj Gabriel, 2013. Used under license from Shutterstock, Inc.

Physician Assistant

A physician assistant (PA) performs many of the duties of a physician, but works under the supervision of the physician. PAs can diagnose and treat illnesses, prescribe medication and provide some treatments. In some rural settings they are the clinical person that a patient may see on a regular basis, when a physician is not available more than one to two days per week. The scope of a PA's prerogatives and duties varies by state, but can be relatively wide. They perform many of the same duties as a nurse practitioner, but the two professions are not the same and should not be confused. The settings for the PA include hospitals and clinics as well the home.

In order to enter a PA program, an undergraduate degree is usually required in addition to experience in the health professions. Most PAs come into the field with experience as emergency medical technicians, paramedics, or in another health profession. Entering a PA program with only volunteer experience is less common, although it does occur. As with many other health professions, the specific undergraduate major is not as important as is the preparation for the program, and it is important for the prospective student to review the requirements of any program in which he/she may be interested. Once in a program, the student can expect to take courses in anatomy and physiology, pathology, diagnosis, and numerous courses specific to the profession. There will also be supervised clinical training and rotations in areas such as internal medicine, emergency medicine, and pediatrics. Specialization is possible for PA training, but is often done following the basic education and certification either on-the-job, or through specialized training.

The field of PA is expected to grow, along with all health professions, and the outlook is bright for employment. Entry level salaries for PAs are in the range of $60,000–$70,000 with a median pay of approximately $86,000 (Bureau of Labor Statistics; www.salary.com). Physician assistants are represented by the American Academy of Physician Assistants (AAPA), and students should be familiar with the organization if they are interested in PA as a career.

Medicine

Physicians diagnose and treat illnesses of all sorts. They are the primary person with the ultimate responsibility for patient care. There are many types of physicians including allopathic (MD), osteopathic (DO), chiropractic (DC), and naturopathic (ND). Each has a defined scope of practice, and all can involve exercise and sport medicine to a certain extent. In addition, a broad list of specialties are available within allopathic and osteopathic medicine, ranging from primary and family care to neurology and surgery. While exercise science has not always been thought of as a typical undergraduate major for entry into medical training, the number of exercise science majors entering medical school has increased and will be likely to continue to do so in the future.

Medical training varies with the type of degree, but typically includes a four-year degree following a bachelor's degree. In addition, several years of internship and residency usually follows the medical degree. The requirements for entry into programs typically include general biology and anatomy and physiology, chemistry through biochemistry, and physics. In addition, aspiring medical students generally must take the Medical College Admission Test (MCAT). The student is encouraged to explore the specific schools of interest well before application deadlines to make sure of the requirements for specific programs. Many universities have specialized advisement centers or advisors for pre-medical students since the preparation for a career in medicine is relatively complicated and difficult to navigate without assistance.

For information on specific areas of practice a student should go to the organizations that represent the various fields:

Allopathic medicine	American Medical Association	http://www.ama-assn.org/ama
Osteopathic medicine	American Osteopathic Association	http://www.osteopathic.org
Chiropractic medicine	American Chiropractic Association	http://www.acatoday.org
Naturopathic medicine	American Association of Naturopathic Physicians	http://naturopathic.org
Podiatric medicine	American Podiatric Medical Association	http://www.apma.org/

Other Health Care Fields

Students with degrees in exercise science are also generally well prepared for other health care fields, such as respiratory therapy, cardiac imaging, and prosthetics and orthotics. Many of these fields require only a year of post-baccalaureate training.

Advanced Training (M.S. or Ph.D) in Exercise Science

For those whose interest in exercise science goes beyond getting a bachelor's degree, and for whom exploring the field in depth within a focused area sounds appealing, a master's or doctoral degree in exercise science is an option to consider. As seen in this book, there are many subfields within exercise science, and each can be studied at the graduate level. With a graduate degree in exercise science, one can pursue careers in many of the same health-related areas as with a bachelor's degree, if the appropriate post-graduate training is taken. One can also embark on a teaching career at the community college or university level. Most community colleges require a master's degree in the content area to teach, and many universities also have teaching positions for those possessing a master's degree. To enter a tenure-track position at a university, a doctoral degree in the discipline is usually required. In certain areas, such as biomechanics and occupational physiology, there are also many opportunities for employment in the corporate sector for people with advanced training in the specialty fields.

In order to gain admission to a graduate program in exercise science, typically an undergraduate degree in exercise science is a prerequisite, but not always. Students potentially interested in this avenue for study should decide in what area they are most interested and apply to programs that have an emphasis and reputation in that area. The American College of Sports Medicine has lists of graduate programs and areas in which they specialize in most areas of exercise science. For students specifically interested in sport and exercise psychology and related areas such as motor behavior, the North American Society for the Psychology of Sport and Physical Activity (NASPSPA) is a good source for graduate programs, as is the American Society of Biomechanics (ASB) for those interested in functional anatomy and biomechanics as a career.

Summary

There are many career possibilities for students in exercise science. Some require extensive training beyond the bachelor's degree while others rely on on-the-job training. It is important to prepare oneself for the career path of choice, which means taking the appropriate classes as an undergraduate, doing volunteer, paid or internship work or other preparation, and maintain a GPE that will ensure competitiveness for the chosen program. It may also be important to have "fall-back" plans in case you either change your mind about the career path you have chosen, or are unable to get into a training program in the chosen field.

References

American Academy of Physician Assistants. http://www.aapa.org/

American Occupational Therapy Association. http://www.aota.org/

American Physical Therapy Association. http://www.apta.org/

Baicker, K., D. Cutler, and Z. Song. 2010. "Workplace Wellness Programs Can Generate Savings." *Health Affairs* 29(2):304–11

Bureau of Labor Statistics. http://www.bls.gov/ooh/healthcare

Cardiacrehabilitationsalary.com

Cepa-acsm.org

Money.usnews.com

Princeton Review. Career-Pharmaceutical Sales Representative. http://www .princetonreview.com/careers.aspx?cid=110

Salary.com

Simplyhired.com